Imaging of Bone and Soft Tissue Tumors

Springer

Berlin
Heidelberg
New York
Barcelona
Hong Kong
London
Milan
Paris
Singapore
Tokyo

T. Rand
P. Ritschl
S. Trattnig
M. Breitenseher
H. Imhof
D. Resnick

Imaging of Bone and Soft Tissue Tumors

A Case Study Approach

With Contributions by
A. Zembsch T. Bindeus M. Kaderk S. Spitz

With 87 Figures in 172 Separate Illustrations

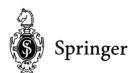

Springer

ISBN 3-540-65096-2 Springer-Verlag Berlin Heidelberg New York

CIP Data applied for

Die Deutsche Bibliothek – CIP-Einheitsaufnahme
Imaging of bone and soft tissue tumors: a case study approach /
T. Rand ... With contributions by A. Zembsch ... – Berlin ; Heidelberg ; New York ;
Barcelona ; Hong Kong ; London ; Milan ; Paris ; Singapore ; Tokyo : Springer, 2001
ISBN 3-540-65096-2

Springer-Verlag Berlin Heidelberg New York
a member of BertelsmannSpringer Science+Business Media GmbH

http://www.springer.de

Cover design: E. Kirchner, Heidelberg
Typesetting: Fotosatz-Service Köhler GmbH, Würzburg

SPIN 10688096   21/3130/op 5 4 3 2 1 0

Preface

The accurate diagnosis of tumors and tumor-like lesions of bones and soft tissues is often challenging, owing in part to the large number of such lesions and their shared clinical manifestations. In the past, imaging of these tumors and tumor-like lesions was frequently limited to conventional radiography. In recent years, however, the application of more advanced imaging methods, especially CT and MR, to the analysis of these lesions has become commonplace. Thus, the physician evaluating these tumors must become familiar with their manifestations in images derived from both conventional and advanced techniques.

This book utilizes individual, carefully chosen cases to emphasize the important imaging characteristics of a variety of significant tumors and tumor-like lesions of bone and soft tissue. The organization of each case includes a short clinical history, several figures that document the routine radiographic, CT and/or MR imaging features of the lesion, a discussion of the differential diagnostic considerations, the rationale for choosing the single most likely diagnosis, a description of the pathologic findings, and a few general comments regarding the specific disease entity. This format makes for easy and enjoyable reading and, further, allows the reader to test his or her knowledge of imaging findings in each individual case. This format is similar to that practiced at the viewbox or console each day at teaching centers throughout the world. It is a tested and effective method of instruction.

The accurate diagnosis of tumors and tumor-like lesions of bones and soft tissues based on clinical and imaging data will clearly remain challenging for years to come. The authors believe, however, that this text provides practical and useful information that, when learned, will make such correct diagnosis possible and even more likely. It is for this reason that the book was written.

Donald Resnick, M.D.
Professor of Radiology, University of California, San Diego

About this Book

This book is out of real life and reflects our traditional Thursday afternoon orthopedic-radiologic conferences, where difficult or questionable cases were discussed among orthopedic surgeons and radiologists. The presentation and analysis of the cases is therefore authentic.

Following the conferences, all patients were operated on at the Orthopedic Hospital Gersthof, Vienna, by Prof. Ritschl's team. Histologic examination was conducted in all cases by the staff of the Department of Pathology of the General Hospital of Vienna (AKH), headed by Prof. Kerjaschki. The work on this book further documents the strong relationship between the osteoradiologic section of Vienna University and Prof. Resnick's legendary "bone pit" at the Veterans Administration Medical Center in San Diego, California.

How to Read this Book

The 39 cases in this book represent osteologic tumors or tumor-like lesions and are presented in random order. The description of each case guides the reader through a virtual discussion with the orthopedic surgeon, starting with the history and continuing with the inspection and analysis of images, the building up of differential diagnoses, and their discussion. The diagnoses vary from classic and easy cases to rare or unexpected solutions – just like in real life.

This book can be read in many ways. The classic way and the one recommended by the authors is to tackle the pages in sequence:

- Page 1 of each case provides the reader with general information.
- Page 2 shows a representative selection of images.
- On page 3 the radiologist gives his differential diagnoses. At the bottom of this page the reader should stop and consider his diagnosis before turning over. This is the time when the radiologist sits in front of the screen and says nothing, while the orthopedic surgeon waits for the diagnosis. It is the critical part of the interaction, with expectations on the one hand and knowledge, originality, wisdom or smartness on the other.
- Page 4 reveals the final diagnosis and further some general aspects of the disease together with useful remarks from the orthopedic viewpoint.

Nevertheless, all other styles of reading – starting with the diagnosis and then viewing the picture; discussing first and then looking for the history; analyzing the images without giving a diagnosis; crying out the diagnosis after having seen the first image; and so on – are allowed. The book will then be an even more realistic reflection of osteoradiologic analytic work!

Contents

Authors and Contributors

Authors

Breitenseher, Martin, M.D.
Professor of Radiology
University of Vienna, Department of Radiology
Waehringer Guertel 18–20, 1090 Vienna, Austria

Imhof, Herwig, M.D.
Professor of Radiology
University of Vienna, Department of Radiology
Waehringer Guertel 18–20, 1090 Vienna, Austria

Rand, Thomas, M.D.
Professor of Radiology
University of Vienna, Department of Radiology
Waehringer Guertel 18–20, 1090 Vienna, Austria

Resnick, Donald, M.D.
Professor of Radiology
University of California, San Diego
Veterans Administration Medical Center
3350 La Jolla Village Drive
San Diego, CA 92161, USA

Ritschl, Peter, M.D.
Professor of Orthopedic Surgery
Orthopedic Hospital Gersthof
Wielemansgasse 28, 1180 Vienna, Austria

Trattnig, Siegfried, M.D.
Professor of Radiology
University of Vienna, Department of Radiology
Waehringer Guertel 18–20, 1090 Vienna, Austria

Contributors

Bindeus, Tanja, M.D.V.
Clinic of Orthopaedics in Ungulates
University for Veterinary Medicine
Veterinärplatz 1, 1210 Vienna, Austria

Kaderk, Monika
University of Vienna, Department of Radiology
Waehringer Guertel 18–20, 1090 Vienna, Austria

Spitz, Sonja, M.D.
Orthopedic Hospital Gersthof
Wielemansgasse 28, 1180 Vienna, Austria

Zembsch, Alexander, M.D.
Orthopedic Hospital Gersthof
Wielemansgasse 28, 1180 Vienna, Austria

Case 1   Hip Joint

History

After suffering pain in both hips for several months this 54-year-old man was referred to the orthopedic surgeon and a plain radiograph was performed. Blood tests revealed no abnormality.

Imaging

1. Plain Film Radiographs

Fig. 1.1
Right hip in abduction, a. p. projection

In the right femoral head and neck region, involving the inferior portion and extending to the central fovea of the femoral head, an ovoid lytic lesion with a partly sclerotic border, in particular involving the superior and lateral cortex can be seen. The lesion is mostly sharply delineated; however, the border to the trochanteric region is less well defined. There is no significant space-occupying effect, and despite the proximity to the cortex no cortical destruction or periosteal reaction can be seen. No intralesion calcification is present. The joint space is unremarkable. Altogether, it seems to be a benign lesion.

2. Magnetic Resonance Imaging

Fig. 1.2
Right hip, coronal plane

a T1-SE
b T1-SE after contrast administration
c STIR

The inferior portion of the right femoral head and neck epimetaphyseal is occupied by a well-defined lesion with diameters of about 6 and 3 cm. On the inferior border a double cortical line is present; however, no significant expansion and no obvious cortical destruction is present. The lesion shows marked hyperintensity on the fat-suppressed sequence (Fig. 1.2c), with a homogeneous appearance. Intralesional septa are present. No perifocal bone marrow edema can be seen. The adjacent soft tissues are unremarkable.
On a T1-weighted spin-echo (SE) sequence the lesion is of hypointense signal intensity and shows moderate, inhomogeneous and lobular appearing contrast enhancement after intravenous contrast media application.
In the superomedial portion of the lesion a metallic artifact after biopsy can be seen.

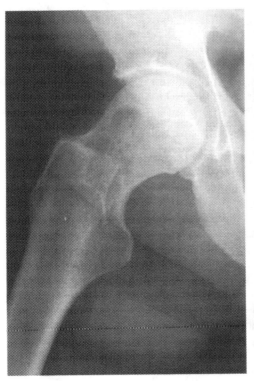
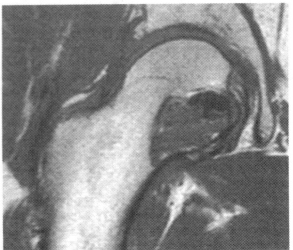
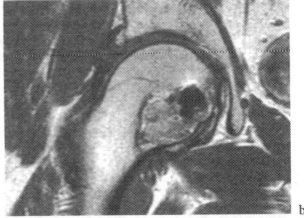
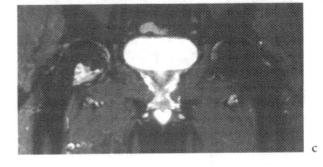

Differential Diagnosis Based on Radiographs

- Giant-cell tumor
- Chondromyxoid fibroma
- Metastases

Differential Diagnosis Based on Radiographs and Further Studies

- Giant-cell tumor
- Benign fibrous histiocytoma
- Chondromyxoid fibroma
- Metastases
- Chondroma
- Fibrous dysplasia

Why and What

1. Giant-Cell Tumor

Giant cell tumor is the most likely diagnosis owing to the localization in the epimetaphyseal region of the bone. Despite the large extension of lucency with a partially ill-defined endosteal margin, no cortical destruction and periosteal reaction can be seen. However, cortical destruction and soft-tissue extension is compatible with giant-cell tumor. Cortical ridges or internal septa produce a multilocular appearance. MRI appearance and contrast enhancement is compatible with giant cell tumor. Typically, no perifocal bone marrow edema is present. The patient's age is atypical (usually 20 – 40 years).

2. Benign Fibrous Histiocytoma

Benign fibrous histiocytoma is benign and somewhat similar to giant-cell tumor.

3. Chondromyxoidfibroma

The predominant localization of a chondromyxoid fibroma is the lower extremity, particularly the tibia in a metadiaphyseal location. Furthermore, T2-weighted MRI usually demonstrates mixed hypointensity, in contrast to the hyperintensity in this case.

4. Fibrous Dysplasia

The homogeneous aspect of the lesion on plain film radiographs and on MRI is atypical for fibrous dysplasia (thick sclerotic border with internal ground-glass appearance, irregular calcifications, and irregular sclerotic areas is typical). Furthermore, no significant expansion is present. Location in the epiphysis is atypical for fibrous dysplasia, which, moreover, is usually diagnosed between 3 and 15 years of age.

5. Metastases

Metastases might demonstrate a more irregular appearance; cortical destruction and potential soft tissue reaction, however, cannot be excluded.

6. Chondroma

Chondroma shows up as a centric lesion with calcifications and a diaphyseal location.

Final Diagnosis

Benign Fibrous Histiocytoma (Benign Variant of Giant-Cell Tumor)

Definition. Benign fibrous histiocytoma is a benign tumor which originates from histiocytes. It is somewhat similar to histiocytic fibroma and giant-cell tumor.

Synonyms. Xanthoma, fibroxanthoma.

Incidence. Very rare.

Age, sex distribution. No gender predilection.

Therapy. Intralesional resection with local adjuvants.

Prognosis. If excision is complete, healing seems to be constant.

Case 2   Ankle

History

This 22-year-old woman had been suffering from pain and swelling of the right heel for 3 months. On clinical examination the patient suffered from minor pain on palpation of the medial calcaneus. Movement in the subtalar joint was painful. At the time of the examination the standard blood tests were negative.

Imaging

1. Plain Film Radiographs

A well-defined extensive bony lesion in the dorsal aspect of the calcaneus adjacent to the tuber calcanei is present. The lesion shows a rim of sclerotic bone and increased lucency in comparison with the normal trabecular bone. No intralesional calcifications can be seen.

2. Magnetic Resonance Imaging

Sagittal T1-weighted sequences reveal a hypointense lesion isointense to muscle in the posterior and medial portion of the calcaneus with a broad contact to the tuber calcanei. After contrast administration homogeneous enhancement can be observed. A thin rim of marked hypointensity representing a sclerotic rim can be seen. On a sagittal STIR sequence there is a marked increase in signal intensity with a fluid-like appearance and several radially oriented and irregularly configured septations within the lesion which remain hypointense. There is a minor expansive tendency of the lesion which is demonstrated at the medial posterior border with thinning of the tuber calcanei and focal convexity of the medial cortical bone of the calcaneus with formation of a neocortex. The same blurred hyperintensity is visible adjacent to the superior cortical border of the calcaneus, including the retrocalcaneal bursa, which is fluid-filled, and inferiorly adjacent to the posterior plantar muscles including the insertion site of the plantar aponeurosis. The fat-suppressed sequences show perifocal bone marrow edema with sparing of the most anterior portion of the calcaneus. In addition, the soft tissue within the tarsal tunnel demonstrates an inhomogeneous increase in signal intensity with less well defined borders. The maximal diameter of the bony lesion is 3.5 cm.

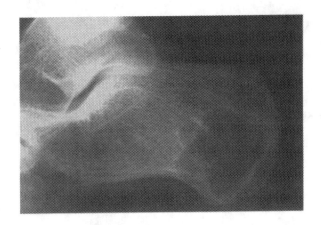

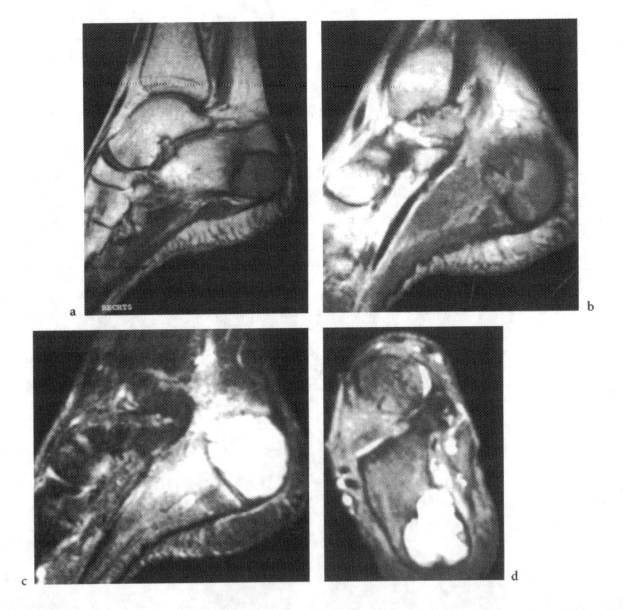

Why and What

1. Aneurysmal Bone Cyst

Eccentric localization, expansion and well-defined lucency with thin, but intact cortex on plain films is typical for aneurysmal bone cyst. Moreover, 70% of such lesions occur in patients less than 20 years old (range: 10–30 years). Furthermore, thin internal strands of bone and new bone in the angle between the original cortex and the expanded part are present. On MRI the signal intensity is more solid than fluid-like, and no fluid-fluid levels are present, which are typical, although not pathognomonic, for aneurysmal bone cyst. Further uncommon are the perifocal bone marrow edema and the reactive edema of the adjacent soft tissues.

2. Simple Juvenile Bone Cyst

A well-defined lytic lesion in the calcaneus without calcification, particularly in a young patient, is a simple cyst until proven otherwise. Hypointense signal on a T1-weighted sequence and hyperintense signal on a T2-weighted sequence with septations are typical. These areas of hypointensity are not true septations but rather ridging on the inner surface of the cyst wall. However, surrounding bone marrow edema and associated soft tissue reaction are not found with simple bone cyst. Moreover, simple bone cysts occur between the ages of 3 and 14 years (mean 9 years) and a male to female ratio of 3:1 is reported.

3. Giant-Cell Tumor

Giant cell tumor presents as a lytic expansive lesion on plain film radiographs with epi- and apophyseal location, compatible with this case. In addition, the age of the patient is typical.
However, giant-cell tumor demonstrates homogeneous contrast enhancement, in contrast to the cystic lesion in this case.

4. Telangiectatic Osteosarcoma

Telangiectatic osteosarcoma is a cystic variant of osteogenic sarcoma. Perifocal bone marrow edema is common; however, the localization and the sclerotic rim of the lesion with a small zone of transition to normal bone is rather atypical for telangiectatic osteosarcoma. In addition, no cortical destruction, periosteal reaction, or soft tissue mass is present, despite the size of the bony lesion. However, telangiectatic osteogenic sarcoma as well as the clear-cell variant of chondrosarcoma may undergo secondary aneurysmal bone cyst formation.

5. Clear-Cell Chondrosarcoma

The clear-cell variant of chondrosarcoma may be cystic; however, the localization, the age of the patient, the well-defined character of the lesion without endosteal cortical thickening or destruction, and the absence of amorphous or punctate calcification make the diagnosis of clear-cell chondrosarcoma very unlikely.

Final Diagnosis

Aneurysmal Bone Cyst with Predominant Solid Variant

Definition. Aneurysmal bone cyst is a pseudotumoral lesion of the bone. It may arise "de novo" in bone where a definite preexisting lesion cannot be demonstrated in the tissue. Secondary forms similar to an aneurysmal bone cyst can be found in various benign conditions and even, rarely, in malignant tumors. The cause of the lesion is unknown.

Incidence. Aneurysmal bone cyst occurs infrequently. Generally it is half as common as giant-cell tumor.

Age, sex distribution. There is a slight predilection for females; the male to female ratio 0.8:1.
Aneurysmal bone cysts occur predominantly (70%) between the ages of 10 and 20 years (70%), although they can be observed at any age.

Location. Aneurysmal bone cysts are found in all portions of the skeleton. The region of the knee, the proximal femur, and the vertebral column are mainly affected. In the vertebral column aneurysmal bone cysts tend to involve the posterior elements.

Therapy. Intralesional resection of the aneurysmal bone cyst associated with the use of local adjuvants (phenol, liquid nitrogen, cement) and bone grafting is the most common treatment modality. In favorable sites, segmental resections (ribs) are performed. In unfavorable sites such as the vertebral column and the pelvis, selective arterial embolization, single or repeated, is used successfully.

Prognosis. The prognosis is excellent. An aneurysmal bone cyst nearly always heals. The recurrence rate after incomplete curettage is 10–15%.

Case 3   Hip Joint

History

This 18-year-old female patient had suffered from repetitive pain in the right hip during movement for 6 months. Clinical examination was normal; standard blood tests were negative at the time of examination.

Imaging

1. Plain Film Radiographs

Fig. 3.1
Right hip joint,
a. p. projection

Plain film radiographs reveal an ovoid geographic lucency in the right intertrochanteric region, with most of the lesion located in the trochanter major area. The maximal diameter is about 3 cm. The lesion shows a bilobar configuration and most of its margin is well defined, although the inferior border reveals a broader zone of transition to the surrounding normal trabecular bone. There is an impression of ground-glass opacity within the lucency; however, no intralesional septa or matrix calcification are present. At the trochanter major the lesion is immediately adjacent to the cortical bone. No cortical destruction or periosteal reaction is present. In addition, minimal expansion of the lesion compared with the contralateral side can be seen in the axial view. The right hip joint is unremarkable.

2. Magnetic Resonance Imaging

Fig. 3.2
Both hips, coronal
plane
a T1-SE
b T1-SE after contrast
administration
c STIR

A coronal T1-weighted SE sequence shows an ovoid lesion with dimensions of about 3.5 by 2.5 cm and with lower signal intensity than the normal bone marrow, but slightly higher signal intensity than the muscles. Intralesional foci of hypointense signal intensity can be seen. After i. v. administration of contrast medium these foci remain hypointense, in contrast to the moderate contrast enhancement of most of the lesion. On a fat-suppressed STIR sequence an intense increase in signal intensity can be seen; however, an inhomogeneous, multilobular appearance is obvious. This lesion is well defined, but surrounded by a large area of low signal intensity on the T1-weighted SE sequence and of marked hyperintensity on the STIR sequence which comprises the femoral neck and the proximal metaphyseal region of the femur including the metadiaphyseal area. The femur epiphysis shows normal signal intensity. The lesion demonstrates minimal expansion and the cortical bone is preserved; however, on the dorsal aspect the lesion is adjacent to the cortex, which appears thinned. No extraosseous soft tissue tumor can be seen.

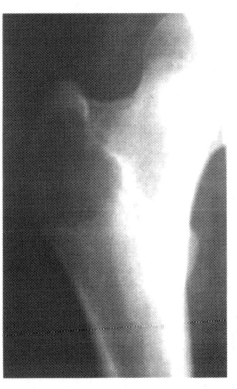

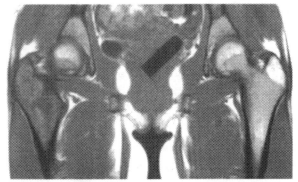
a

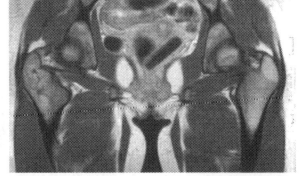
b

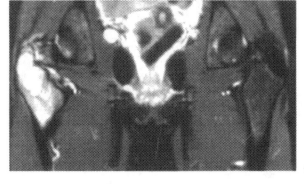
c

Differential Diagnosis Based on Radiographs

- Chondroblastoma
- Aneurysmal bone cyst
- Giant-cell tumor
- Eosinophilic granuloma

Differential Diagnosis Based on Radiographs and Further Studies

- Giant-cell tumor
- Chondroblastoma
- Eosinophilic granuloma

Why and What

1. Giant-Cell Tumor

Localization (apophysis) of a long bone and the finding of a lucency with an at least partially ill-defined endosteal margin on plain film radiographs and a multilocular appearance with nearly homogeneous contrast medium uptake on MRI (STIR sequence) is compatible with giant-cell tumor. However giant-cell tumors are more typically found in middle age. Aggressive behavior of the tumor with perilesional bone marrow edema can be seen with higher grades of giant-cell tumor.

2. Chondroblastoma

Lesion localization and age of the patient are rather typical for chondroblastoma (age: 5–20 years; 50% occur in the lower limb in epi- or apophyseal location). However, on plain film radiographs the typical well-defined lucency with a sclerotic rim and internal calcifications is not present.

On MRI chondroblastoma can sometimes be distinguished from giant-cell tumor by intravenous administration of Gd-DTPA, since the chondromatous matrix of chondroblastoma takes up less contrast medium and usually perifocal edema is more prominent than in giant-cell tumors. However, chondroblastomas may also demonstrate high vascularity, and perifocal edema can also be observed in giant-cell tumors.

Both entities are located epi- or apophyseally; however, the latter has its epicenter in the metaphysis and secondarily involves the epiphysis, occurring after plate closure.

3. Eosinophilic Granuloma

Typically this lesion appears in younger subjects (4–7 years) and the child presents with bone pain, local swelling, and irritability. The lucency is usually well defined, and endosteal scalloping may be seen as well as a sclerotic rim. On MRI perifocal bone marrow edema and contrast medium uptake is typical. Localization in the apophysis is uncommon.

4. Aneurysmal Cyst

Localization, expansion, and mostly well-defined lucency on plain film is typical for aneurysmal bone cyst. Moreover, 80% of such cysts occur in patients less than 20 years of age (range 10–30 years).

However, on MRI no fluid-like lesion is present, the lesion is solid and takes up contrast medium. Additionally, perifocal bone marrow edema as well as reactive edema of the adjacent soft tissue is uncommon in aneurysmal bone cysts.

Final Diagnosis

Giant-Cell Tumor, Grade 2 (Moderate Proliferation)

Definition. The exact cell of origin of this neoplasm is still unknown. The multinucleated giant cells apparently result from fusion of the proliferating mononuclear cells, which are most probably of histiocytic origin. The giant cells are a constant and characteristic element of this neoplastic proliferation. This differentiates this tumor from numerous other skeletal lesions where the giant cells constitute occasional reactive elements. The giant-cell tumor presents a distinct clinical, topographical, and radiographical entity.

Incidence. Giant-cell tumor occurs relatively frequently.

Age, sex distribution. There is a slight predilection for females. The peak incidence is in the 3rd decade of life. Over 80% of the neoplasms occurs in patients over 20 years of age. The observation of giant-cell tumor prior to puberty is exceptional. The tumor is also rarely observed over the age of 50 years.

Location. Approximately 90% of giant-cell tumors are observed in metaepiphyseal and metaapophyseal regions of long bones, nearly 45% are located at the knee region. Further sites are the distal radius, the proximal femur, the distal tibia, and the proximal humerus. Also the sacrum and the pelvis can be affected, as well as the vertebral bodies.

Therapy. Intralesional resection using an adequate window in the bony wall as well as local adjuvants such as phenol is the treatment of choice. The reconstruction is achieved by bone grafting. In advanced cases marginal or wide excisions have to be performed. In these cases reconstruction is carried out using autogenous materials or allografts. In rare cases en bloc resection and a tumor endoprosthesis are necessary.

Prognosis. The local recurrence rate has been reported to be about 50% after intralesional resections. With modern therapeutic modalities such as chemical and thermal cautery, however, the figure should be approximately 20%. The recurrence usually occurs within 2 years of treatment, although it has also been seen even after 7 years. In rare cases a benign giant-cell tumor can metastasize singly or multiply to the lungs.

Case 4   Knee

History

This 57-year-old patient had suffered from intermittent pain of the right knee joint for several months. A 3- to 5-cm lesion was palpable on the ventromedial joint compartment in the region of the pes anserinus. The lesion was non-movable and painless. The lesion further revealed no signs of inflammation, and no varices were evident.

Imaging

Fig. 4.1
Right knee

a A.p. projection
b Lateral projection

1. Plain Film Radiographs

The plain film radiographs show no abnormality.

2. Magnetic Resonance Imaging

Fig. 4.2
Right knee

a T1-SE after contrast administration, sagittal plane
b T1-SE after contrast administration, axial plane
c T2-SE, sagittal plane

At the level of the tibial condyle on the medial and dorsal aspects a well-defined cystic lesion can be identified. The lesion lies ventral to the medial head of the gastrocnemius muscle and is separated from the muscle by a thin line of fatty tissue on all sections. The cystic lesion appears to consist of two portions, each measure about 1.5 cm in maximal diameter, with the sartorius muscle tendon running between them. Superiorly both cystic lesions seem to communicate and measure up to about 3 cm in maximal diameter. At this level a tubular extension runs parallel to the posterior cortex of the medial tibial condyle and anteriorly to the tendon of the semimembranosus tendon. Furthermore, this tubular extension seems to be in contact with the posterior horn of the medial meniscus. The semitendinosus tendon runs adjacent to the lateral border of the lesion. After intravenous administration of contrast medium no solid tumor formation can be demonstrated. The wall is thin and septations are present.

The posterior horn of the medial meniscal is reduced in volume and appears partially hyperintense on T1-weighted sequences.

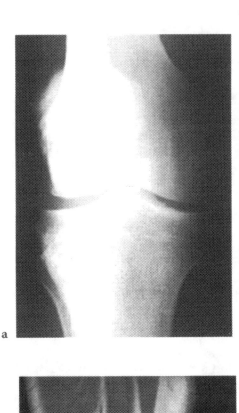

a

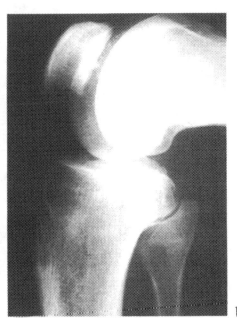

b

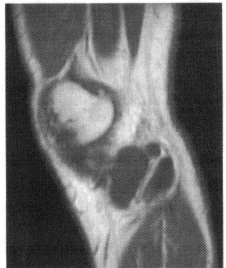

a

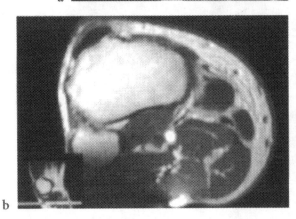

b

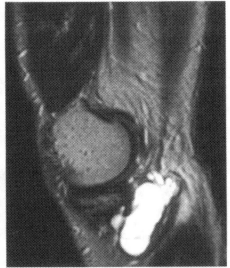

c

Why and What

1. Pes Anserinus Bursitis
Masses along the medial joint line with the signal characteristics of water on all pulse sequences can be due to bursitis or bursal enlargement, ganglia, and meniscal cysts. The multilobulated cystic lesion in this case, which ensheaths the linear hypointense pes anserinus (semimembranosus, semitendinosus, and sartorius tendon complex), and projects exactly along the course of the pes anserinus complex, not above or below it, as do most Baker cysts, is compatible with pes anserinus bursitis. However, the lack of tenderness of the lesion does not support an inflammatory condition.

2. Meniscus Ganglion
Ganglia communicate with the joint space but not with the menisci and invariably align themselves with tendons. Meniscal cysts communicate with the menisci and are associated with meniscal tears. Communication of the cystic lesion with the meniscus is suggested on the axial and sagittal images. Although close contiguity with the pes anserinus tendons is suggested in the sagittal projection, communication with meniscus would be unusual in association with pes anserinus bursitis or Baker cyst and is far more likely to occur with meniscal cysts.

3. Atypical Baker Cysts
The anatomic location in the axial plane is atypical for popliteal cysts, since these cysts arise from the posterior medial horn of the gastrocnemius-semitendinosus bursa in 90 % of cases. The mass in this case lies medial and anterior to the bursal interface. In 10 % of cases the location of a Baker cyst is atypical, which may show a communication with the joint cavity; however, communication with the medial meniscus is not expected.

4. Varicous Disease
The location, morphology, and signal intensity, as well the lack of contrast enhancement, are inappropriate for varices.

Final Diagnosis

Parameniscal Ganglion

Definition. Superficially located mucoid lesion. The ganglion originates from a mucoid transformation in situ of the connective tissue.

Synonym. Mucous cyst.

Incidence. Frequent.

Age, sex distribution. Most common between 25 and 45 years of age. No gender predilection.

Location. Predilection for the periphery of the meniscii of the knee.

Therapy. Surgical removal.

Prognosis. Good; local recurrence may occur after incomplete resection.

Case 5   Femur

History

This obese 22-year-old woman had suffered from unspecific knee pain for a period of 12 months. She had had several courses of antiinflammatory treatment and had consulted various physicians. Because of a growing mass in the popliteal region, radiographs were obtained.

Imaging

1. Plain Film Radiographs

Fig. 5.1
Distal right femur in lateral projection

The main pathological feature is a tumor mass attached to the dorsal aspect of the distal femur. The cortical bone in this area is eroded and partially destroyed. In the lateral view the tumor seems to invade the medullary canal. The ventral corticalis is intact, although there is a periosteal reaction in this area. The tumor mass shows popcorn like calcification.

2. Computed Tomography

Fig. 5.2
Distal right femur, axial plane and bone window

The tumor mass itself shows multiple small and cloudy mineralizations. The cortical bone is widened; the corticalis is destroyed in the posterior aspect.

3. Magnetic Resonance Imaging

Fig. 5.3
Distal right femur

a T1-SE images, coronal plane
b T1-weighted SE after contrast administration, sagittal plane
c T1-weighted SE after contrast administration, axial plane

Magnetic resonance imaging of the right distal femur demonstrates a mass at the level of the diametaphysis. The intraosseous part of the mass has a size of 4 × 3 cm; on the dorsal side a big soft tissue mass measuring 12 × 6 × 6 cm is seen. This lesion is of low and rather homogeneous signal intensity in the T1-weighted spin-echo sequence (Fig. 5.3a). After intravenous administration of contrast medium, strong and inhomogeneous enhancement can be seen. Moreover, multiple dots of low signal intensity are found in all parts of this soft tissue tumor (Figs. 5.3b, c). The tumor itself looks septated and lobulated. The intraosseous as well as the soft tissue part of the tumor is well delineated from the surrounding bone marrow, fatty tissue, and muscles. Though there is very close proximity between the dorsal tumor margin, the vessels, and the nerve, no sign of infiltration is seen (Fig. 5.3c).

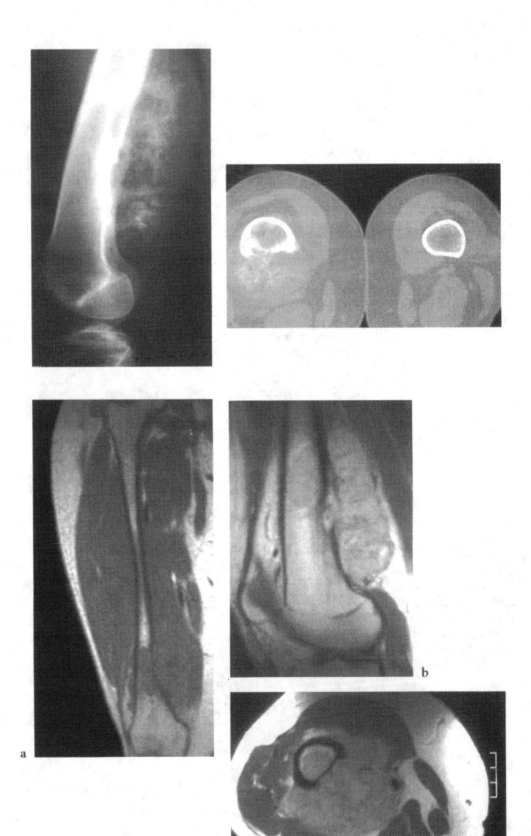

Differential Diagnosis Based on Radiographs

- Chondrosarcoma
- Parosteal osteosarcoma

Differential Diagnosis Based on Radiographs and Further Studies

- Parosteal osteosarcoma
- Chondrosarcoma
- Mesenchymal chondrosarcoma

Why and What

1. Chondrosarcoma

The pattern of calcification within the osseous and soft tissue components of this lesion is stippled, similar to that of a chondrosarcoma. In fact, all of the roentgenographic abnormalities resemble those of a typical chondrosarcoma. It is the relatively young age of the patient that may allow a diagnosis of atypical chondrosarcoma. The MR findings speak against a chondrosarcoma because of the homogeneous and strong contrast enhancement.

2. Osteosarcoma

The patient's age, the parosteal location, and the MRI findings are more characteristic for the presence of an osteosarcoma, especially since the small calcifications cannot be differentiated on MRI. However, radiographs demonstrate rather clear calcifications of a chondromatous matrix.

3. Mesenchymal Chondrosarcoma

The divergence between radiographs, indicating a chondromatous tumor, and the MR images, indicating an osseous tumor, leads to the suspicion of a mesenchymal chondrosarcoma. Although relatively rare, mesenchymal chondrosarcoma is one of the few primary malignant tumors of bone that not infrequently arises in the soft tissues. Patients with mesenchymal chondrosarcoma typically are younger than those with conventional chondrosarcoma and similar in age to those with conventional osteosarcoma. The pattern of calcification within the osseous or soft tissue component of the lesion usually is stippled, similar to that of a conventional chondrosarcoma.

As the radiographic findings of mesenchymal chondrosarcoma are those of an aggressive tumor that contains calcification, it generally is not possible to differentiate this neoplasm from a conventional chondrosarcoma. The fact that mesenchymal chondrosarcomas are observed in relatively young patients assumes some diagnostic importance.

Final Diagnosis

Mesenchymal Chondrosarcoma

Definition. The tumor is characterized by a bimorphic pattern:
- Highly undifferentiated small round cells with some slight spindling quality.
- Chondroid components of variable size which are usually well differentiated or look benign.

Incidence. Rare in the soft tissues and even rarer in the skeleton.

Age, sex distribution. Observed during young adult hand, age from 15 to 40 years. There is no gender predilection.

Location. Everywhere in the skeleton, preferably in the neck and lower limbs.

Therapy. Wide or radical surgical removal. The effectiveness of chemo- or radiotherapy is not proven.

Prognosis. Most cases have a fatal outcome.

Case 6   Knee

History

This 14-year-old boy complained of pain and swelling in the distal left femur. Additional symptoms and signs included an increase in local skin temperature and restriction of movement in the adjacent articulation.

Imaging

1. Plain Film Radiographs

Fig. 6.1
Left knee, a. p. projection

The radiograph of the left knee reveals an eccentric osteolytic lesion involving the metaphyseal segment of the distal left femur, with osseous expansion, trabeculation, and periosteal reaction. This lesion is enclosed by a shell of bone. The inner margin of the lesion is well defined with a rim of bone sclerosis, and the cortical surface of the affected bone is expanded or ballooned. There is no adjacent soft tissue mass.

2. Magnetic Resonance Imaging

Fig. 6.2
Left knee

a Coronal T1-SE after contrast administration
b Axial T1-SE after contrast administration with fat presaturation
c Coronal T2-weighted sequence with fat suppression (STIR)

On T1-weighted images the lesion is well defined and demonstrates low signal intensity. A cortical bowing is seen in a low signal intensity; the contour of cortical bone is intact. The contrast medium sequences demonstrate a small marginal area of intraosseous enhancement with periosteal as well as soft tissue enhancement which is inhomogeneous and of irregular border but without a clear mass effect (Figs. 6.2a, b). Coronal T2-weighted MR images with fat suppression show an expansive lesion of inhomogeneous but mainly high signal intensity with internal septation of low signal intensity (Fig. 6.2c).

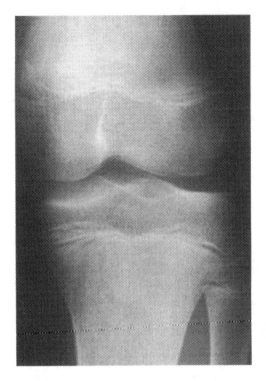

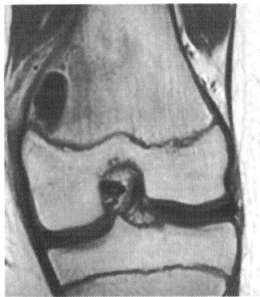

a

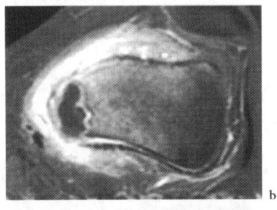

b

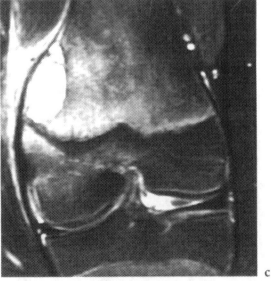

c

Why and What

1. Aneurysmal Bone Cysts

The imaging features suggest the diagnosis of an aneurysmal bone cyst because of the patient's age, the eccentric metaphyseal location in the distal femur, the cystic and aneurysmatic character on radiographs, and the fluid-containing, only marginally enhancing lesion on MRI. Additionally, a periosteal reaction and edema of soft tissue and bone marrow can be observed on MRI.

Aneurysmal bone cysts are usually observed in the first, second, or third decade of life. They are most frequent in the long tubular bones and the spine. Within the long tubular bones, aneurysmal bone cysts are seen predominantly in the metaphysis.

An expansive and lobulated or septated lesion is typical. The internal septations create cystic cavities whose walls contain diverticulum-like projections. A thin, well-defined rim of low signal intensity around an aneurysmal bone cyst is common. The signal intensity characteristics within this rim are variable. Although high signal intensity commonly is evident in parts of an aneurysmal bone cyst on T2-weighted SE MRI, it is not present uniformly.

Fluid levels also may be identified. Such levels are not diagnostic for an aneurysmal bone cyst and occur also in giant-cell tumors, simple bone cysts, chondroblastomas, and telangiectatic osteosarcoma. Nevertheless, they are most compatible with the diagnosis of aneurysmal bone cyst.

2. Enchondroma

Enchondroma is less expansive, contains calcifications, and is mainly located in the center of the long bones. It is rarely seen in eccentric location.

3. Nonossifying Fibroma

The metaphyseal and cortical locations on the distal femur in the second decade are consistent with the diagnosis of a nonossifying fibroma, but otherwise lead one to expect a less expansive and non aggressive appearance without a periosteal reaction and more sclerosis.

4. Giant-Cell Tumor (Giant Cell Reparative Granuloma)

Giant-cell tumor is most common in the epiphyseal location with solid and contrast-enhancing tumor parts, which are not present in this case.

5. (Telangiectatic) Osteosarcoma, Ewing Sarcoma

A more aggressive and destructive pattern with solid intraosseous tumor and soft tissue tumor, typical with this diagnosis, is not present in this case.

6. Inflammation

The adjacent bone marrow and soft tissue should demonstrate more reactive changes for this diagnosis.

Final Diagnosis

Aneurysmal Bone Cyst

Definition. Aneurysmal bone cyst is a pseudotumoral lesion of the bone. It may arise de novo in bone where a definite preexisting lesion cannot be demonstrated in the tissue. On the other hand, areas similar to an aneurysmal bone cyst can be found in various benign conditions and even, rarely, in malignant tumors. The cause of the lesion is unknown.

Incidence. Aneurysmal bone cyst occurs infrequently. Generally it is half as common as giant-cell tumor.

Age, sex distribution. Aneurysmal bone cysts occur predominantly (70%) between the ages of from 10 and 20 years, although they can be observed at any age. There is a slight predilection for females: male to female ratio 0.8:1.

Location. Aneurysmal bone cysts are found in all portions of the skeleton. The region around the knee and the proximal femur, as well as the vertebral column, are mainly affected. In the vertebral column aneurysmal bone cysts tend to involve the posterior elements.

Therapy. Intralesional resection associated with the use of local adjuvants (phenol, liquid nitrogen, cement) and bone grafting is the most common treatment modality. In suitable sites segmental resections are performed.
In unfavourable sites such as the vertebral column and the pelvis, selective arterial embolization, single or repeated, is successful.

Prognosis. The prognosis is excellent. Aneurysmal bone cysts nearly always heal. The recurrence rate after incomplete curettage is 10–15%.

Case 7

Ankle, Distal Lower Leg

History

Two months after the birth of this boy the parents recognized an asymmetry of the lower extremity which was pronounced at the medial ankle. The boy was seen by an orthopedic surgeon at the age of 1 year. At this time palpation revealed a nondefined mass. The skin around the swelling was flexible and normothermic.

Imaging

1. Plain Film Radiographs

Fig. 7.1
Both ankles,
a. p. projection

Plain radiographs of the ankles on both sides in a.p. projection show marked tissue swelling in the region of the medial ankle of the left side compared with the other side. There is no evidence of osseous deformity.

2. Magnetic Resonance Imaging

Fig. 7.2

a. Left ankle and distal lower thigh, T1-SE, coronal plane
b Left ankle and distal lower thigh, T1-SE, sagittal plane
c Left ankle, T2-SE with fat suppression (STIR), axial plane

Magnetic resonance imaging performed at the age of 10 months revealed in-homogeneous formations in the subcutaneous fat of the left shank extending to the soft tissues of the medial ankle with a partly serpiginous appearance (Figs. 7.2a, b). On axial T2-weighted images with fat suppression the area demonstrates punctate high signal intensity. The mass is adjacent to the tibia over a long distance, but there is no evidence of osseous destruction. Muscles are not infiltrated. There is little fluid in the joint.

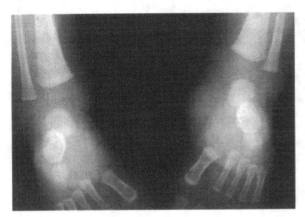

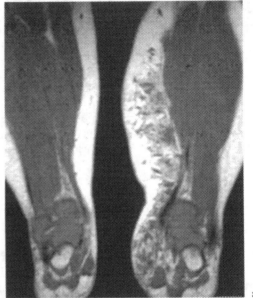

a

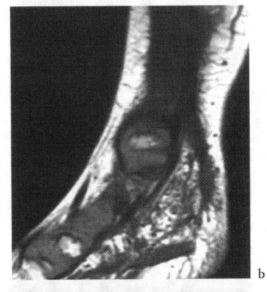

b

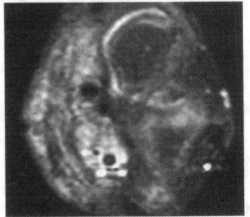

c

Why and What

1. Lymphangioma

This tumor consists of a proliferation of lymphatic vessels and belongs to the group of angiomatoses. These lesions are typically poorly marginated and isointense relative to skeletal muscles on T1-weighted MR images. Within the lesions there might be bands that contain areas with high signal intensity identical to that of fat. On T2-weighted images lymphangiomas are better marginated and hyperintense compared with subcutaneous fat, but they may also contain segments that are isointense relative to fat or muscle.

2. Hemangioma

Radiographs of hemangiomas may reveal evidence of soft tissue masses containing circular calcified collections termed phleboliths. In addition, osseous involvement, overgrowth and articular abnormalities, especially in the knee due to accompanying synovial lesions, may be encountered. Angiography may allow precise documentation of the pattern of vascular proliferation; however, tubular appearance of signal alterations indicates a vascular nature of the lesion.

3. Angiosarcoma

Angiosarcomas are rare malignant tumors of the soft tissues, comprising less than 1% of sarcomas. These lesions are classified according to the dominant cell type. A tumor composed of lymphatic endothelioblasts is termed lymphangiosarcoma. It may affect various parenchymas (bones, liver, breast), the soft tissues, or the skin. In the latter case it may be associated with lymphedema. Onset in the arm is typical with postmastectomy lymphedema. Lymphangiosarcoma less commonly complicates congenital, traumatic, or idiopathic lymphedema. Since onset of the malignant neoplasm on a preexisting lymphangiomatosis has been reported in a few cases, angiosarcoma cannot be excluded from the differential diagnosis in this case.

Final Diagnosis

Lymphangioma of the Limbs

Definition. It is often difficult to state whether lymphangiomas are true neo-plasms, harmatomas or lymphangiectasias. Most authors regard lymphangiomas as malformations, arising from sequestration of lymphatic tissue that failed to communicate normally with the lymphatic system. They accumulate vast amounts of fluid, which accounts for their cystic appearance.

Incidence. Compared with hemangiomas, lymphangiomas are relatively rare. Bill Sumna counted five cases among 3000 admissions of children to ortho-pedic hospitals.

Age, sex distribution. Of these tumors, 50–65% are present at birth and 90% are manifest by the end of the 2nd year of life. Those which are present dur-ing adult life are superficial cutaneous lymphangiomas. Sex distribution is roughly equal.

Location. Lymphangiomas affect almost any part of the body but show a predilection for the head, neck and axilla. They also can occur in parenchymal organs including the gastrointestinal tract, spleen, liver and bone. In associa-tion with hemangiomas it is called Maffucci syndrome.

Therapy. Although rare cases of spontaneous regression have been reported, all lesions require surgical treatment. The extent of the procedure is dictated by the location and the desire to achieve reasonable cosmetic results. For pa-tients presenting lesions early in life the suggested time for surgery is between the ages of 18 and 24 months.

Prognosis. Although lymphangioma is a benign lesion it may cause significant morbidity because of its large size, critical location and the possibility of sec-ondary infection. Usually cystic lymphangiomas are well circumscribed and more amenable to complete excision. Local recurrence may occur. Sclerosing agents and radiotherapy have been employed in the past but should not be used as alternatives to surgery. Irradiated lymphangiomas may transform to an malignant tumor.

Remarks

As opposed to most cases of lymphangiomatosis, which usually have exten-sive visceral involvement associated with a very poor prognosis, involvement in this variant is limited almost exclusively to the soft tissues of the limb and the prognosis is good. The soft tissue lesions may be associated with involve-ment of the adjacent bones. A specific diagnosis can be provided by lymph-angiography owing to the accumulation of the contrast material in the intra-osseous lymphangiomas. This finding suggests the possibility that lymphan-giomas of the bone are produced by insuffiency and agenesis of the valves within dysplastic subcutaneous lymph vessels that lead to lymphatic back flow into bone.

Case 8 — Distal Femur

History

This 27-year-old woman presented with recurrent pain in the distal third of the left thigh. Palpation revealed an area of indolent hard popliteal resistance, approximately 10 cm in diameter just above the knee joint. The skin was flexible and normal. No sign of additional vascularization (or venous hypervascularization) was noted. Flexion of the knee joint was dolent and incomplete due to the supraarticular dorsal mass. At the time of examination the standard blood tests were negative.

Imaging

1. Plain Film Radiographs

Fig. 8.1
Distal femur

a Lateral projection
b Enlargement of the cortical lesion

Plain film radiographs reveal an irregularity of the dorsal aspect of the femoral cortex and a lucent area centrally metadiaphyseally (Fig. 8.1). The lucency measures about 3 × 4 cm. Additionally soft tissue swelling adjacent to the dorsal aspect of the femur has to be suspected.

2. Computed Tomography

Fig. 8.2
Distal femur, axial plane, bone window

Computed tomography reveals an adherent osteolytic lesion, 3 cm in diameter, within the central part of the femur condyle approximately 2 cm above the knee joint (Fig. 8.2). This lytic lesion destroys the dorsal corticalis and has an extension towards the medial femur condyle, which shows cortical thinning. The cranio caudal extension of the tumor is 8.5 cm within the medullary cavity of the femur. The rather large extraosseous soft tissue component extends dorsally along the dorsal border of the femur and infiltrates the dorsal upper thigh musculature. This soft tissue part of the tumor appears rather inhomogeneous, especially after administration of contrast medium, and shows centrally regressive parts (with liquid attenuation).
On the CT images no articular involvement can be seen.

3. Magnetic Resonance Imaging

Fig. 8.3
Distal femur

a T1-SE, sagittal plane
b T1-SE after contrast administration, sagittal plane
c T2-SE, sagittal plane

A large mass with hypointense signal on T1-SE images can be seen with intra- and extramedullary extension of the tumor (Fig. 8.3a). After contrast medium administration there is inhomogeneous enhancement, with some central parts remaining hypointense (Fig. 8.3b). On T2-SE images most of the extramedullary part of the tumor remains hypointense with only some small central liquid formations (Fig. 8.3c). A slight increase of synovial fluid within the knee joint can be seen as well (articular effusion). There is surrounding bone marrow edema within the right femur.
Invasion of the biceps muscle can be seen on MRI. Also an invasion into the knee joint at the insertion of the anterior cruciate ligament has to be suspected on MRI, as the upper insertion of the cruciate ligament appears rather inhomogeneous; no bony structures can be discerned between the tumor mass and the insertion of the anterior cruciate ligament.

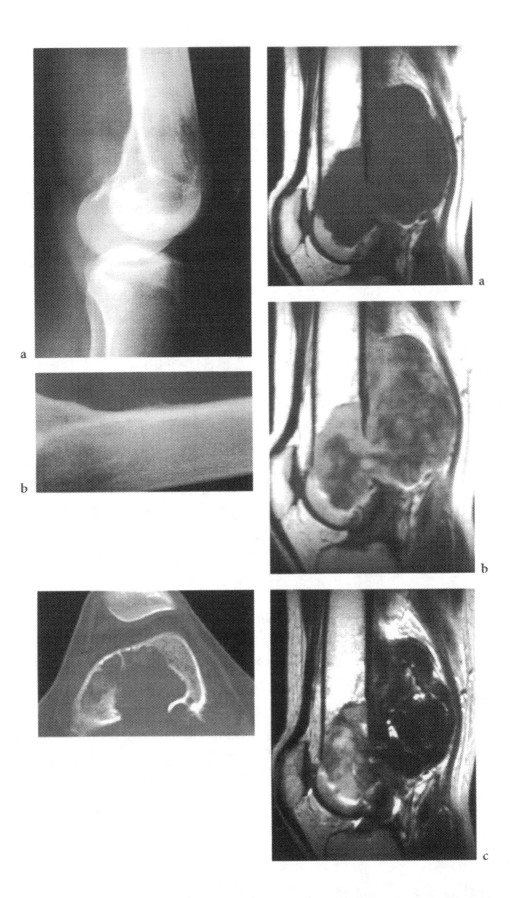

Why and What

1. Osteosarcoma
The rather inhomogeneous appearance of the tumor with typical intense contrast medium enhancement and intra- and extraosseous components, as well as the age of the patient, are consistent with the diagnosis of osteosarcoma. In a patient of appropriate age, osteosarcoma is always the first differential diagnosis. Due to the regressive areas within the tumor, indicating fast growth, malignancy is assumed.

2. Malignant Fibrous Histiocytoma
Generally malignant fibrohistiocytoma (MFH) originates in the medial dorsal condyle of the femur and is a rather slow growing tumor without a large extraosseous component. Therefore, the appearance of the tumor makes MFH very unlikely.

3. Lymphoma
Generally, lymphoma can be used as a differential diagnosis for any musculoskeletal tumor. Usually the regressive changes within the tumor are not as extensive as in this case. On the other hand, the polygonal appearance of the tumor makes lymphoma, which is usually intramedullary, rather unlikely.

4. Soft Tissue Sarcoma Infiltrating Bone
Osseous infiltration of soft tissue surrounding the bone can also appear in a primary soft tissue mass. However, in this case the tumor seems to grow out of the bone into the soft tissue, and also the intraosseous component seems to be too large for a primary soft tissue mass.

5. Chondrosarcoma
Chondrosarcomas typically display coarse calcifications, but neither on CT nor on MRI is these any hint of calcifications. Therefore, chondrosarcoma can be excluded.

Final Diagnosis

Fibroplastic Intermediate Grade Osteosarcoma (II)

Definition. Osteosarcoma is a neoplasm with proliferating malignant cells which produces an osteoid matrix. Osteoid, chondroid or fibromatoid differentiation may be predominant.

Incidence. Except for myeloma, osteosarcoma is the most common primary bone tumor. Its incidence is about 4–6 cases per 1 million per year.

Age, sex distribution. Seventy-five percent of all cases become manifest between 10 and 30 years of age. The peak incidence is in the second decade. There is a predilection for males, with a sex ratio of 1.5–2:1.

Location. Metaphysis of long bones, especially the distal and proximal femur, proximal humerus and proximal tibia.

Therapy. The treatment of osteosarcoma consists of chemotherapy and wide or radical surgical excision. Radiotherapy is generally not used. After biopsy, preoperative chemotherapy is performed. The definitive surgical procedure is generally conducted 10 weeks after the biopsy. After the surgery an adjuvant chemotherapy is carried out.

Prognosis. The survival rate with surgical treatment alone was 10–20%. Generally pulmonary metastases occurred within 1–2 years after amputation. Nowadays these figures have changed drastically, so that the 5-year survival rate after chemotherapy is approximately 60–70%. The response to chemotherapy is the single most important prognostic factor. When the tumor necrosis exceed more than 90%, the outcome is good in more than 80% of the cases. Other factors influencing the prognosis are the size and site of the tumor.

Remarks

For the orthopedic surgeon it is important to know whether the lesion has an intraarticular component or not. The intramedullary and/or extraosseous part of the tumor and its relationship to the surrounding tissue have further effects on the surgical management and therefore have to be reported in great detail. The relationship to the popliteal vessels and nerve structures is important. Tumor invasion into the popliteal vein should be reported. Always include a "long fat-saturated inversion recovery sequence" of both the whole femora and the adjacent tibiae to exclude skip lesions.

Case 9   Knee

History

After a trauma this patient complained of pain, swelling, and inflammation of the right knee joint. Leukocytes and sedimentation rate were elevated. After puncture of the knee joint a yellowish joint effusion was found.

Imaging

1. Plain Film Radiographs

Fig. 9.1
Right knee,
a. p. projection

Plain film radiographs demonstrate a 3-cm osteolytic lesion in the center of the proximal epiphysis of the tibia adjacent to the subchondral bone (Fig. 9.1). The border of this lesion shows a sclerotic rim without destruction of the surrounding bone. No matrix calcification can be obtained. The knee joint itself has many signs of osteoarthritis.

2. Magnetic Resonance Imaging

Fig. 9.2
Right knee

a Proton-density dual
T2-TSE, sagittal plane
b DESS-3D-GE, sagittal
plane
c T2-GE, coronal plane

Magnetic resonance imaging demonstrates a cystic lesion in the proximal epiphysis of the tibia. The lesion is well delineated and has a sharp border; it is lobulated and demonstrates septations. The border of the lesion is of low signal intensity in all sequences with sclerotic rim. Perifocally no bone marrow edema or infiltration of the surrounding bone marrow is observed. The lesion is of inhomogeneous and low signal intensity in the proton-density dual T2-turbo spin-echo (TSE) sequence (Fig. 9.2a) and of intermediate to high signal intensity in the DESS-3D-gradient-echo (GE) sequence (Fig. 9.2b). The T2-weighted sequences reveals an onion-like structure. An additional finding can be obtained in coronal images in the area of the intercondylar eminence where a minute duct seems to connect the lesion with the knee joint. The knee joint itself demonstrates a large joint effusion and signs of osteoarthritis with cartilage thinning and subchondral sclerosis.

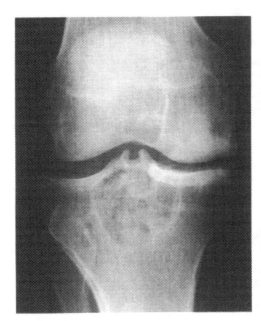
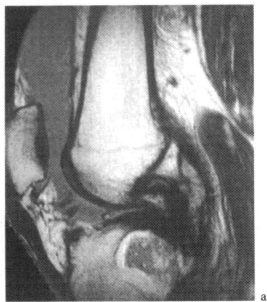
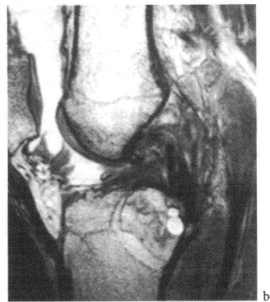
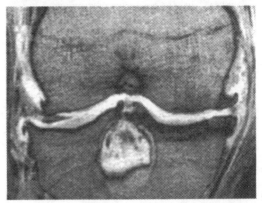

a

b

c

Differential Diagnosis Based on Radiographs

– Giant-cell tumor
– Simple bone cyst
– Cyst associated
  with degenerative
  joint disease
– Chondroblastoma

Differential Diagnosis Based on Radiographs and Further Studies

– Intraosseous ganglion
– Giant-cell tumor or
  benign fibrous histio-
  cytoma

Why and What

1. Intraosseous Ganglion

The diagnosis of intraosseous ganglion is most likely, owing to the bony and soft tissue connections to the knee joint and the high signal intensity on the T2-weighted sequence. Furthermore, the lobulated and subseptated border of the lesion is compatible with an intraosseous variant of a ganglion. There is no evidence of biological activity or tumor growth, as no perifocal bone marrow edema can be obtained.

2. Giant-Cell Tumor

Giant-cell tumor is a differential diagnosis from plain film radiographs, where the finding is a well-defined lucency. On MRI a giant-cell tumor should demonstrate a high and more homogeneous signal intensity on T2-weighted sequences and sometimes shows a perifocal bone marrow edema, depending on tumor growth. Further, the sclerotic rim is thinner without the lobulations and subseptations found in this case. Nevertheless, localization in the epiphysis and in the proximal tibia is typical for a giant-cell tumor.

3. Others

With combined evaluation of radiographs and MRI, further differential diagnoses can be excluded. There is no tumor matrix calcification consistent with chondroblastoma. Furthermore, there is no general homogeneous low signal intensity in T2-weighted sequences, as in tumors containing more fibrous tissue.

Final Diagnosis

Intraosseous Ganglion

Definition. Intraosseous ganglion develops within the bone in the proximity of a joint. The differential diagnosis includes cysts associated with degenerative joint disease. The anatomopathological nature of these cysts is the same as that of the more well known and common ganglions of the soft tissue.

Synonyms. Ganglion of bone, subchondral or juxtaarticular bone cyst, synovial cyst of bone.

Incidence. Intraosseous ganglions are seen occasionally.

Age, sex distribution. The lesion is observed during adulthood. There is a predilection for males, with a sex ratio of 1.5 : 1.

Location. The ankle, the knee and the hip region, as well as the wrist, are mainly affected. Generally the ganglion is located in the vicinity of a joint surface.

Therapy. Intralesional resection and packing of the cavity with bone chips.

Prognosis. In exceptional cases there may be a recurrence, even when the excision was complete, owing to mucoid transformation of the surrounding connective tissue.

Case 10   Finger

History

This 60-years-old woman presented with a 6-month history of a slowly increasing, painless swelling at the palmar aspect of the proximal phalanx of the fifth digit. On palpation the lesion was hard.

Imaging

1. Plain Film Radiographs

Fig. 10.1
Fifth digit

a A.p. projection
b Lateral projection

Radiographs demonstrate a soft tissue swelling of the proximal phalanx of the fifth finger without soft tissue calcification and without destruction or reaction of the bone (Fig. 10.1).

2. Magnetic Resonance Imaging

Fig. 10.2
Fifth digit

a T2-SE, sagittal plane
b T2-SE with fat suppression (STIR), sagittal plane
c T1-SE after contrast administration with fat suppression, axial plane

Magnetic resonance reveals a soft tissue mass $7 \times 10 \times 20$ mm in size. The border of the tumor is well circumscribed. The signal intensity is high in T1-weighted images, intermediate in T2-weighted images (Fig. 10.2a) and decreased in fat-suppressed images (Fig. 10.2b). After administration of contrast medium, no signal increase can be observed. The lesion is in broad contact with the flexor tendon sheath, and there is no evidence of bone invasion.

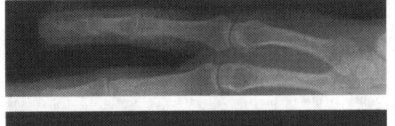

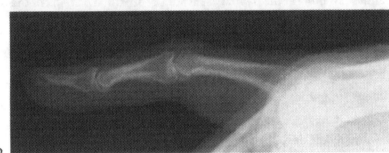

◄

Fig. 10.1. Fifth digit

a A.p. projection
b Lateral projection

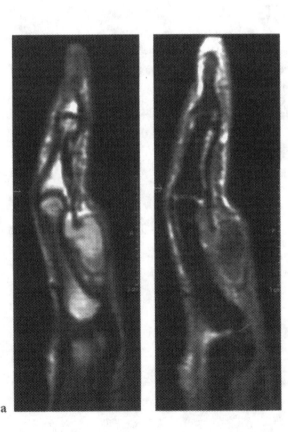

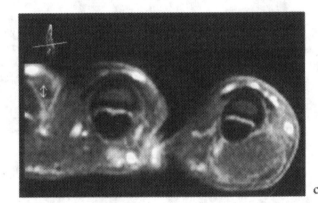

Fig. 10.2. Fifth digit

a T2-SE, sagittal plane
b T2-SE with fat suppression (STIR), sagittal plane
c T1-SE after contrast administration with fat suppression, axial plane

Why and What

In contrary to plain film radiographs, which are rather unspecific, MRI findings are almost specific in this case, owing to the signal characteristics in individual sequences.

1. Lipoma

This diagnosis is considered due to the lesions, high signal on T1 weighting with signal decrease in fat-suppressed images and lack of contrast enhancement.

Other differential diagnoses can be discussed only theoretically:

2. Liposarcoma

For a liposarcoma more contrast enhancement whould be expected.

3. Synovialoma

Location and configuration are consistent with synovialoma. Presence of fat in small parts of a synovialoma is possible. However, the large extent of fat signal and the low contrast enhancement in this case is incompatible with the diagnosis of synovialoma.

4. Giant-Cell Tumor of the Tendon Sheath

The location of the tumor with a broad contact to the flexor tendon might suggest giant-cell tumor as a potential diagnosis; however, the signal intensities, indicating high fat content, and the lack of contrast enhancement do not indicate this tumor.

Final Diagnosis

Lipoma

Definition. Solitary lipomas consist entirely of mature fat. Lipomas are occasionally altered by the admixture of other mesenchymal elements. The most common of these structures is fibrous connective tissue, often hyalinized, which may or may not be associated with a capsule or fibrous septa.

Incidence. The reported incidence of lipoma is probably much lower than the actual incidence. Nevertheless, it represents the most common neoplasm of mesenchymal origin.

Age, sex distribution. Lipomas are rare during the first two decades of life. They appear mainly in the fifth and the sixth decade. Some authors report a higher incidence in men, others in women.

Location. Two types of solitary lipoma are distinguished:

1. The superficial type is most common in the region of the back, shoulder, upper neck, and abdomen, followed by the proximal portions of the extremities.
2. Deep-seated lipomas are rare in comparison. They are found in the mediastinum, the retroperitoneum, the chest wall, and the extremities.

Therapy. Marginal excision is the treatment of choice.

Prognosis. Lipomas are benign. They may recur locally after intralesional resection. Malignant transormation is extremely rare.

Case 11 Elbow

History

This 58-year-old man observed a slowly growing mass in the proximal fore-arm anteriorly, with pain on movement, over a period of 3 months. No history of trauma was reported. On clinical examination a well-circumscribed flexible mass could be palpated in the area of the antecubital fossa.

Imaging

1. Plain Film Radiographs

Fig. 11.1
Left elbow, lateral
projection

A lateral radiograph of the elbow demonstrates almost normal bone structures. Only a small exostosis at the proximal radius on the insertion point of the biceps tendon can be seen. No soft tissue calcification is present. An ill-defined soft tissue swelling can be discerned at the level of the forearm muscles near the elbow joint.

2. Magnetic Resonance Imaging

Fig. 11.2
Left elbow

a T1-SE, sagittal plane
b T2-SE, sagittal plane
c T1-SE after contrast
administration, sagittal
plane

Magnetic resonance imaging of the left elbow demonstrates a soft tissue mass in the proximal forearm. This mass shows low and rather homogeneous signal intensity on T1-weighted images (Fig. 11.2a). T2-weighted images demonstrate areas from very low through intermediate to high signal intensity (Fig. 11.2b). After intravenous administration of gadolinium, intermediate to high uptake can be observed (Fig. 11.2c). The margin of the lesion is irregular. At the proximal side there is contact with the capsule of the elbow joint. No infiltration of the muscles or subcutaneous fat is present. The cortical bone and bone marrow are not invaded.

Within the lesion in an eccentric position a band-like and in all sequences hypointense structure can be seen which seems to be in continuity with the biceps tendon. The tendon itself shows clearly alterations with increased signal intensities on the T1- and T2-weighted sequences, an irregular appearance, and a thickened diameter.

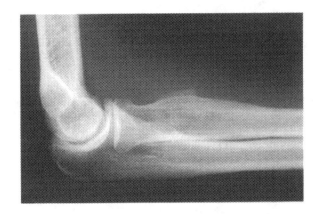

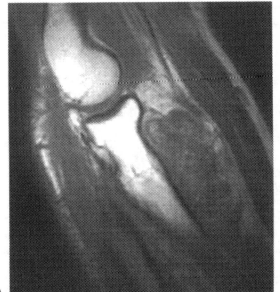

a

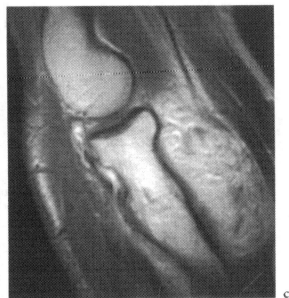

c

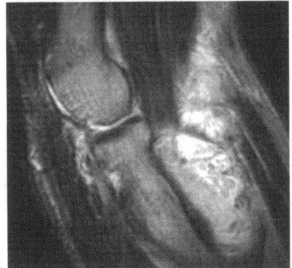

b

Why and What

1. Tendinous Pseudotumor

The combination of the changes in the biceps tendon with the mass or mass-like lesion at the distal insertion side is rather indicative of tendinous pseudotumor. Thickening and signal alteration of this biceps tendon suggests a subacute or chronic rupture. Tendon ruptures are associated with peritendinous changes from a soft tissue edema to a chronic, mass like inflammation on the base of a healing reaction.

Normal tendons appear as smooth, linear structures of low signal intensity on MRI. Tendinous tears, partial or complete, are associated with irregular and frayed contours and alterations in signal intensity of the tendon. Complete tears are accompanied by discontinuity and retraction of the tendon. The alteration in signal intensity depends on the age of the injury. Obliteration of nearby fat planes and hematomas are also seen. With healing, scar formation develops in the injured tendon that may lead to regions of low to intermediate signal intensity and also contrast enhancement.

2. Soft Tissue Tumor

The imaging features might suggest a soft tissue tumor. Lipomatous tumors or vascular tumors can be excluded due to the absence of characteristic signal intensities of fat or vascular structures. The relation to the biceps tendon might indicate a synovial or tendinous origin.

3. Synovial Sarcoma

Synovial sarcoma is a clinically and morphologically well-defined malignant tumor of the soft tissue. It is located most frequently in the soft tissue of the extremities. The neoplasms generally arise adjacent to a joint, bursa, or tendon sheath. Synovial sarcomas occur at all ages but are most frequent in the young adult. The tumor is mostly solid with necrotic areas, signs of infiltration, destruction, or displacement. In this case the tumor looks less aggressive, but a synovial sarcoma cannot be excluded with confidence.

4. Pigmented Villonodular Synovitis

Pigmented villonodular synovitis usually demonstrates lower signal intensity on T2-weighted images owing to hemosiderin deposition in 50% of cases, and mostly shows lower uptake of contrast medium, combined with cortical erosions, signs which are not present in this case.

Final Diagnosis

Chronic Complete Rupture of the Biceps Tendon at the Bony Insertion

Definition. Avulsions and tears of tendons around the elbow are most frequently a consequence of physical injury. The rupture of the distal portion of the tendon of the biceps brachii muscle is rare, constituting less than 5% of all biceps tendon injuries. The typical mechanism of the injury is forceful hyperextension applied to a flexed and supinated forearm.

Incidence. Rare.

Age, sex distribution. This lesion generally occurs in men after 40 years of age and in the dominant arm.

Location. Although rupture of the distal portion of the tendon of the biceps brachii muscle is rare, it represents an important injury of the elbow, most frequent in the dominant extremity.

Therapy. Adhesiolysis and refixation of the tendon.

Case 12   Thumb

History

This 15-year-old girl presented with an increasing painless, circumscribed swelling at the apex of the left thumb.

Imaging

1. Plain Film Radiographs

Fig. 12.1
Thumb

a A.p. projection
b Lateral projection

Plain film radiographs reveal a small soft tissue swelling without matrix calcification and without thinning or bowing of the adjacent cortical bone at the apex of the left thumb.

2. Magnetic Resonance Imaging

Fig. 12.2
Right thumb

a T1-SE, coronal plane
b T2-weighted inversion recovery sequence with fat suppression (STIR), coronal plane
c T1-SE with fat presatu-ration and after contrast administration (SPIR), axial plane

Magnetic resonance imaging of the left thumb reveals a small soft tissue mass in the apex of the thumb. The lesion is ovoid with a size of 6 × 8 × 10 mm. The lesion demonstrates a sharp border. In the T1-weighted sequence a hypo-intense and thin capsule can be seen (Fig. 12.2a). The center of the lesion is of intermediate signal intensity in this sequence. In the STIR sequence this lesion is overall of high signal intensity, though a minimal signal decrease can be noticed in the center (Fig. 12.2b). After administration of contrast medium an intermediate signal increase is visible. The same sequence with fat presat-uration demonstrates the contrast medium uptake more clearly and precisely, especially in contrast with the surrounding fatty tissue. Again, a subtle signal decrease in the center is obvious (Fig. 12.2c). No infiltration of the surround-ing soft tissue or cortical bone can be observed.

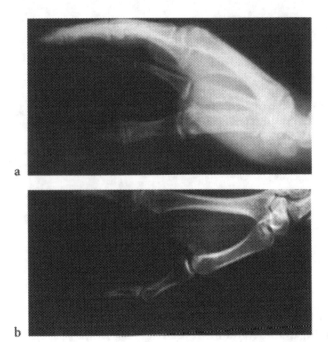

Differential Diagnosis Based on Radiographs

- Inflammation
- Foreign body
- Skin thickening
- Tumor

Differential Diagnosis Based on Radiographs and Further Studies

- Soft tissue tumor with subtle content of fat in the center
- Neurinoma, neuro-fibroma, hemangioma
- Inflammation

Why and What

1. Pseudomass (Inflammation or Granuloma)
Radiographs show a nonspecific thickening of the apex of the thumb. Only a limited number of lesions can be excluded by radiographs, such as lesions based on soft tissue calcifications, e.g., scleroderma and hyperparathyroidism. Furthermore, radiopaque foreign bodies can be excluded.

2. Neurinoma, Neurofibroma
Location, size and contrast medium enhancement are consistent with this diagnosis. Furthermore, the high signal intensity on T1-weighted postcontrast MRI contributes to this diagnosis, though a rather high extent of fat signal is found in this case.

3. Hemangioma
Location, size and signal characteristics with contrast enhancement might suggest a hemangioma. However, additional to the differential diagnosis of a neurofibroma the usual clinical signs and typical tubular structures of hemangioma are absent.

4. Lipoma
Magnetic resonance imaging gives a rather clear impression of a small soft tissue mass with subtle content of fat. Nevertheless, the fat content is too little for the diagnosis of a typical lipoma. In addition, contrast enhancement is atypical for lipoma.

5. Sarcoma
The intermediate and inhomogeneous enhancement after administration of contrast medium supports the idea of a sarcoma. The tumor margins are well defined, but this finding is not important for the differentiation of benign and malignant tumors. Usually the size is an useful indicator of the benign or malignant nature of a soft tissue mass. However, in the present location the lesion need not be large to be malignant. Therefore, the signs of a mass, contrast medium enhancement, and fat content lead us to the diagnosis of liposarcoma.

Final Diagnosis

Low-Grade Liposarcoma

Definition. Liposarcoma is a malignant tumor of the soft tissue with a variable histological picture, ranging from well-differentiated lipoma-like liposarcoma to round-cell liposarcoma, myxoid liposarcoma, and pleomorphic liposarcoma.

Incidence. Between 10% and 12% of all soft-tissue sarcomas.

Age, sex distribution. Liposarcoma is a tumor of adult life, with a peak incidence between 40 and 60 years of age. Very occasionally it occurs in younger patients, particularly in those between 10 and 15 years. Liposarcomas of the limbs show a mild predilection for males.

Location. There is a predilection for deep-seated locations. The most frequent sites are the thigh, particular the quadriceps, and the popliteal region, followed by shoulder and arm. The most frequent site in the trunk is the retroperitoneum.

Therapy. Wide or radical surgical removal is the treatment of choice. Marginal and intralesional excision should be avoided because of the high incidence of local recurrences. Supplementary radiotherapy and chemotherapy are widely performed, especially in pelvic and retroperitoneal liposarcoma. These treatment modalities are widely used in association with surgery.

Prognosis. The histological division of liposarcoma into well-differentiated, myxoid, pleomorphic and round-cell variants is important because of the different courses.
Well-differentiated and myxoid liposarcomas generally have a low grade of malignancy, while pleomorphic and round-cell liposarcoma are characterized by higher-grade malignancy.
The latter type of liposarcoma metastasizes more frequently and relatively early.

Remarks

Occasionally liposarcoma occurs in younger patients, especially between 10 and 15 years of age. In this age group the tumor is generally well differentiated or of the myxoid type.

Case 13   Knee, Distal Femur

History

This 31-year-old woman suffered from pain and swelling in the distal femur and knee joint. No evidence of fever and no trauma were recorded in the history of the patient.

On physical examination no limitation of hip and knee movement was observed. No abnormal neurological findings were present. Standard blood tests were negative

Imaging

1. Plain Film Radiographs

Fig. 13.1
Knee, lateral projection

Soft tissue calcifications can be observed on the medial and dorsal aspect of the distal femur. The calcifications are small, with a cloudy appearance and an overall size of 3 × 7 cm, and they are in connection with the corticalis. The border of the corticalis itself is rather well preserved with the exception of a small circumscribed impression and thinning dorsally with scalloping and remodeling of the adjacent bony cortex.

2. Computed Tomography

Fig. 13.2
Knee, axial plane, bone window

Computed tomography demonstrates a 3 × 7 cm periosteal mass of the distal femur on the dorsomedial aspect. The soft tissue mass is of muscle-like density. The cloudy calcifications are centrally located. Within the extensive contact area with the cortical bone, circumscribed impression and thinning of the cortical bone combined with cortical thickening at the margins can be observed. Irregular cortical thickening can also be seen at the proximal aspect of this lesion.

3. Magnetic Resonance Imaging

Fig. 13.3
Knee

a T1-SE, axial plane
b T2-SE with fat suppression (STIR)

Magnetic resonance imaging reveals a 4 × 6 × 8 cm parosteal mass at the distal femur dorsomedially. The lesion is of low and homogeneous signal intensity in T1-weighted images and of mostly high signal intensity combined with multiple small foci of low signal intensity in T2-weighted images. It is surrounded by a capsule-like structure of decreased signal intensity on T1- and T2-SE images. No infiltration of the muscles can be observed. There is circumscribed and complete destruction of the cortical bone with an extension of about 1.5 × 1.5 cm and with local infiltration of the bone marrow.

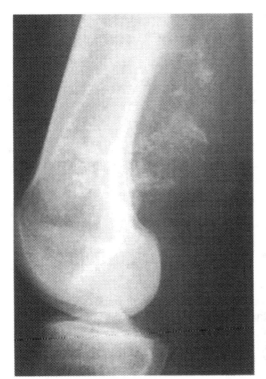

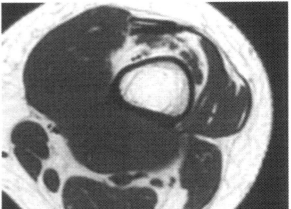

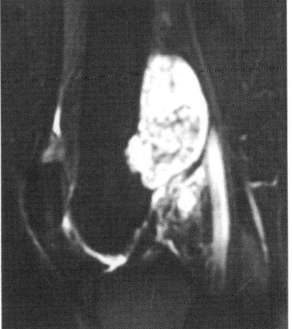

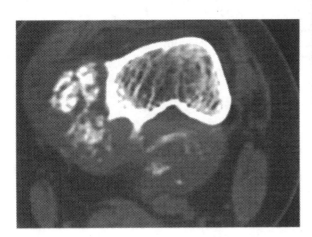

Why and What

1. Parosteal or Juxtacortical Chondrosarcoma

Patients are older and the sarcomas tend to be larger for this diagnosis. The lesion has an aggressive radiologic pattern with cortical destruction and bone marrow involvement. In this case, circumscribed cortical destruction and bone marrow involvement, more evident on MRI than on CT or radiographs, reinforce the suspension of a low grade sarcoma.

2. Parosteal Chondroma

The radiographic features of this lesion include scalloping or remodelling of the adjacent bony cortex and a soft tissue mass with internal calcification. The cloudy calcifications in this case are more typical for a chondromatous than an osseous tumor matrix. Those findings of a parosteal chondroma may recur and sometimes have atypical features, including absence of calcification within the cartilaginous mass and minimal or no erosion of the adjacent cortex. Parosteal or juxtacortical chondroma is an uncommon lesion of bone. There is no sex predilection, and patients' age ranges from 4 to 70 years with an average of 23 years. The lesions occur in the humerus, femur, and fingers. They are metaphyseal, with the majority in the proximal metaphysis. They appear to originate in the periosteum or cortex without evidence of medullary cavity involvement.

3. Parosteal or Periosteal Osteosarcoma

Parosteal osteosarcoma appears as a central ossifying foci with irregular outlines and may be connected to the underlying bone by a stalk. Periosteal osteosarcoma arises in the cortex of the diaphysis of a tubular bone and produces cortical thickening and spiculated osteoid matrix, not present in this case.

4. Myositis Ossificans

Myositis ossificans demonstrates typical calcifications with sharp cortical bone surrounding a lacy pattern of new bone, indicating that maturation proceeds centrifugally, not present in this case. In most cases a radiolucent zone separates the lesion from the underlying cortex. Nevertheless, in the first few weeks calcifications do not present with this typical pattern. Furthermore, a history without recalled trauma does not indicate myositis ossificans.

Final Diagnosis

Parosteal Chondrosarcoma

Definition. Chondrosarcoma which arises from the surface of long bones. The classification as an entity itself is justified by its anatomic and radiographic features and above all the favorable prognosis.

Incidence. Rare.

Age, sex distribution. The tumor is most common at 30–70 years of age. The male:female ratio is 2:1.

Location. Most frequently localized in the metaphysis or towards one end of the diaphysis of long bones such as the femur, tibia, and humerus.

Therapy. Wide resection.

Prognosis. Parosteal chondrosarcoma is much less malignant than central chondrosarcoma of the same histological grade. There is little or no tendency to metastasize.

Case 14   Spine

History

This 58-year-old woman revealed an acute onset of thoracolumbar pain after a chiropractic manipulation during physical therapy. At the time of presentation there was no clinical evidence of a neurologic deficit.

Imaging

1. Plain Film Radiographs

Fig. 14.1
Lumbar spine, lateral projection

Plain radiographs demonstrate marked osteoporosis. The lateral radiograph clearly depicts the vertebral deformity and posterior displacement of a portion of the first lumbar vertebral body into the spinal canal (Fig. 14.1). Additionally, degenerative changes are present.

2. Magnetic Resonance Imaging

Fig. 14.2
Lumbar spine

a T1-SE, sagittal plane
b STIR-SE, sagittal plane
c T2-weighted image with fat suppression (STIR), sagittal plane

The sagittal T1-weighted SE and T2-weighted TSE sequences disclose a homogeneously decreased signal intensity of the bone marrow affecting all vertebral bodies (Figs. 14.2 a – c).
The first lumbar vertebral body is hyperintense compared with the other vertebral bodies on STIR images and demonstrates marked deformity and a loss of height which is most pronounced in the anterior portion (Figs. 14.2 b, c). There is spinal canal stenosis of about 30 % due to posterior displacement of a part of the vertebral body into the canal (Fig. 14.2 c). The dural sac is impressed, but the conus and cauda equina are not affected. There is stripping of the posterior longitudinal ligament from the posterior margin of the vertebral body, which remains intact. No free fragments of bone are present (Fig. 14.2 c). The 12th thoracic vertebral body and the second lumbar vertebral body demonstrate slight signal alteration near the endplate and mild deformity.
There is a focal area of high signal intensity near the endplate of the second lumbar vertebral body on the T1- and T2-weighted SE sequence.

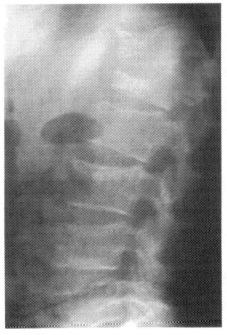

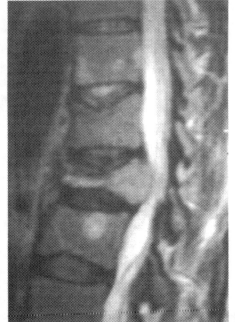

Fig. 14.1. Lumbar spine, lateral projection

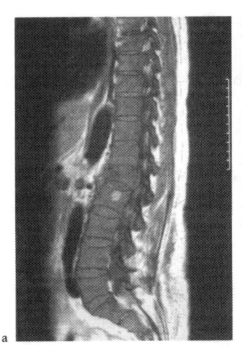

Fig. 14.2. Lumbar spine

a T1-SE, sagittal plane
b STIR-SE, sagittal plane
c T2-weighted image with fat suppression (STIR), sagittal plane

Why and What

1. Hematopoetic Disorders

In patients with leukemia plain films disclose osteoporosis in 60% of cases due to infiltration of the marrow by leukemic cells. Secondary compression fractures can result. Other findings in the spine include lucent bands and multiple focal defects. Osteosclerotic areas are rarely marked. On MRI patients with leukemia demonstrate homogeneously decreased signal on short-TR images (T1-SE) secondary to the replacement of the high-signal fatty marrow by leukemic cells. Foci of leukemic infiltration display increased signal intensity on long-TR images (T2-SE). Although sclerotic foci are rare, they can be seen as regions of low signal intensity on both short- and long-TR images.

2. Secondary Compression Fracture Owing to Metastatic Disease

Metastatic disease, for example in breast carcinoma, can be seen as a diffuse process; however, signal alterations on T1- and T2-weighted sequences are usually inhomogeneous owing to mostly combined osteolytic and osteoblastic disease.

Deformity and high signal alteration of the first lumbar vertebral body on the T2-weighted sequence with height loss is highly suspicious for a recent compression fracture.

3. Osteoporotic Compression Fracture

Osteoporotic spine disease can be excluded since high-signal fatty marrow is replaced by a diffuse process on the T1-weighted SE sequence, indicating infiltrative bone marrow disease.

Final Diagnosis

Secondary Compression Fracture, Hemangioma

Secondary compression fracture of the first lumbar vertebral body with spinal canal narrowing in a patient suffering from acute lymphatic leukemia. Small hemangioma in the second lumbar vertebral body.

Definition. Acute lymphatic leukemia is present if the number of blasts of the bone marrow exceeds 30% of all nucleus-containing cells (morphological criteria of the French-American classification). Leukemias are divided into acute myeloid leukemia (AML), acute lymphatic leukemia (ALL), chronic myeloid leukemia (CML), and chronic lymphatic leukemia (CLL), which is encountered in the low-malignant non-Hodgkin lymphomas.

Incidence. Acute lymphatic leukemia is frequently observed in childhood, before the age of 12. There is a second peak around 65 years of age.

Age, sex distribution. Men are more frequently affected than women (1.5:1). The incidence of manifestation in the second decade is 2 in 100 000 pear year.

Clinical findings. The clinical manifestations are generally directly related to the insufficiency of the bone marrow by elimination of the regular hematopoesis. Anemia, bleeding, thrombocytopenia, and infections result. Extra-skeletal manifestations can affect the skin, lymph nodes, spleen, pericardium, central nervous system, etc.

Therapy. Remission-induction therapy with consolidation and maintenance therapy is administered with the goal of eliminating the leukaemic clone. Combination chemotherapies and early bone marrow transplantation are recommended.

Prognosis. Early therapy in children achieves high remission rates. However, results of therapy in adults are still poor.

Remarks

The typical thoracolumbar compression fracture results in loss of height of the anterior vertebral body with preservation of the middle and posterior spinal columns. In severe compression fractures partial or complete posterior ligamentous injury may be present. The usual treatment for these injuries is conservative. Vertebral compression that leads to loss of more than 40% of the height of the anterior part of the vertebral body often requires posterior stabilization, even in the absence of a neurologic deficit, to prevent progressive spinal deformation.
Note that young children suffering from leukemia – especially those less than 7 years of age – may have a paucity of fat in their bone marrow. In these cases leukemic infiltration may be more difficult to detect.

Case 15   Shoulder

History

This 62-year-old woman with a history of breast carcinoma 10 years earlier suffered from progressive pain in the right shoulder.

Imaging

1. Plain Film Radiographs

Fig. 15.1
Right shoulder,
a. p. projection

Plain film radiograph of the right shoulder in antero-posterior projection reveals a small area of opacification at the greater tuberosity. The lesion is singular, homogeneous and shows no calcifications. No periosteal reaction or soft tissue involvement is observed (Fig. 15.1).

2. Computed Tomography

Fig. 15.2
Right shoulder, axial
plane, bone window

Transverse CT shows a 1.5-cm well-defined homogeneous osteolytic and excentrically located lesion at the greater tuberosity with a sclerotic margin. Calcifications and periosteal reaction are not observed. The cortex is intact; there is no soft tissue involvement (Fig. 15.2).

3. Magnetic Resonance Imaging

Fig. 15.3
Right shoulder

a T1-SE, coronal oblique
plane
b T2-weighted image
with fat suppression
(STIR), coronal oblique
plane

Additionally, partial high signal intensity of the supraspinatus tendon and fluid in the subdeltoid bursa can be observed (Fig. 15.3b), representing degeneration and inflammatory bursal disease.
A small, homogeneous, sharply bordered, low-signal-intensity lesion in the greater tuberosity is demonstrated on the T1-SE image (Fig. 15.3a). The lesion shows high signal intensity on fat-suppressed T2-weighted images (STIR) (Fig. 15.3b). No peripheral edema is seen.

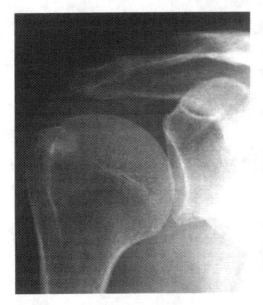

Fig. 15.1. Right shoulder, a. p. projection

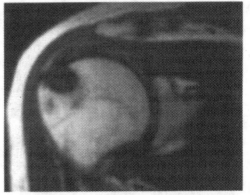

a

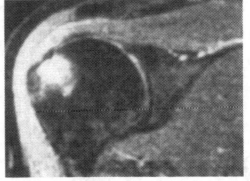

b

Fig. 15.3. Right shoulder

a T1-SE, coronal oblique plane
b T2-weighted image with fat suppression (STIR), coronal oblique plane

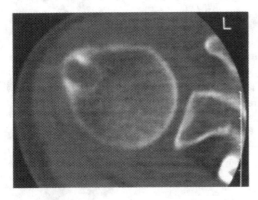

Fig. 15.2. Right shoulder, axial plane, bone window

Why and What

1. Degenerative Sclerotic Cyst by Partial Rotator Cuff Tear

Degenerative changes develop where the tendinous fibers of the rotator cuff attach to the greater tuberosity, most often in the area of the insertion of the supraspinatus tendon. Degenerative cysts and sclerosis of the greater tuberosity can be observed.

2. Reactive Cyst or Pit Formation

Foci of hypointense signal on T1-weighted and hyperintense signal on T2-weighted imaging in a subarticular location contiguous to the promontory insertion of the rotator cuff is compatible with pit formation.

Just as synovial invagination may develop in the hip anterosuperiorly, the so-called herniation pit, so too cyst-like areas may develop in the humerus. These areas almost always occur adjacent to the supraspinatus tendon insertion and are more frequently visualized in athletes. They are not symptomatic but may be associated with tendinitis. However in this case the patient is not an athlete and is older.

3. Enchondroma, Low-Grade Chondrosarcoma

A cystic lesion with a sclerotic rim on radiographs and hyperintense signal on T2-weighted MRI may suggest enchondroma. However, the location is atypical, and neither matrix calcification nor ground-glass appearance is present.

4. Metastasis

In patients with primary cancer a solitary metastatic lesion has to be considered. However, the location at the insertion site of the supraspinatus tendon, the associated changes of tendon and bursa and the peripheral contrast enhancement are much more suggestive of a degenerative cyst.

5. Intraosseous Ganglion

Radiographic and MRI appearance are compatible with intraosseous ganglion; however, the extracapsular location excludes this diagnosis.

Final Diagnosis

Protein-Filled Degenerative Cyst

Definition. Subchondral bone cysts may appear as solitary or multiple lesions of variable size and shape. A cyst implies a cavitary lesion. For a degenerative or osteoarthritic cyst an epithelial lining is not necessary. The cyst may contain proteinaceous material. The probable mechanism of cyst formation is synovial intrusion and bony contusion.

Age, sex distribution. Protein-filled cysts are frequently seen in degenerative cases, generally in older patients. There is no gender predilection.

Location. The pressure segment of subchondral bone.

Therapy. Generally conservative treatment. In the case of persistant pain decompression of the subacromial space may be performed.

Prognosis. Slow progression of the degenerative disease has to be expected.

Case 16　　Proximal Humerus

History

This 43-year-old man reported an 8-month history of pain of the right upper arm. No additional signs were evident.

Imaging

1. Plain Film Radiographs

Plain film radiographs reveal a lytic lesion in a metadiaphyseal location at the proximal humerus with a longitudinal extension of about 6 cm. The borders of the lesion are not well circumscribed; centrally, small popcorn-like calcifications can be seen. Endosteal scalloping is present, and the cortex of the affected bone is moderately thickened. There is no soft tissue involvement or swelling (Fig. 16.1).

2. Computed Tomography

Small calcifications within the lytic lesion can be observed (Fig. 16.2).

3. Magnetic Resonance Imaging

Coronal T1-weighted images reveal a hypointense lesion in the proximal metadiaphyseal part of the humerus with irregular sclerotic margins, a maximal longitudinal extension of 6 cm, and complete infiltration of the medullary cavity (Fig. 16.3 a). The lesion is clearly hyperintense on STIR images with central spotted, small hypointense nodular signal alterations (Fig. 16.3 b).
After administration of contrast medium there is a pattern tiny spotted and septum-like enhancement in the peripheral part of the lesion (Fig. 16.3 c).
A slight endosteal irregularity, but without any defect or interruption of the cortex, can be seen. No periosteal reaction is present, but the affected cortex is moderately thickened.

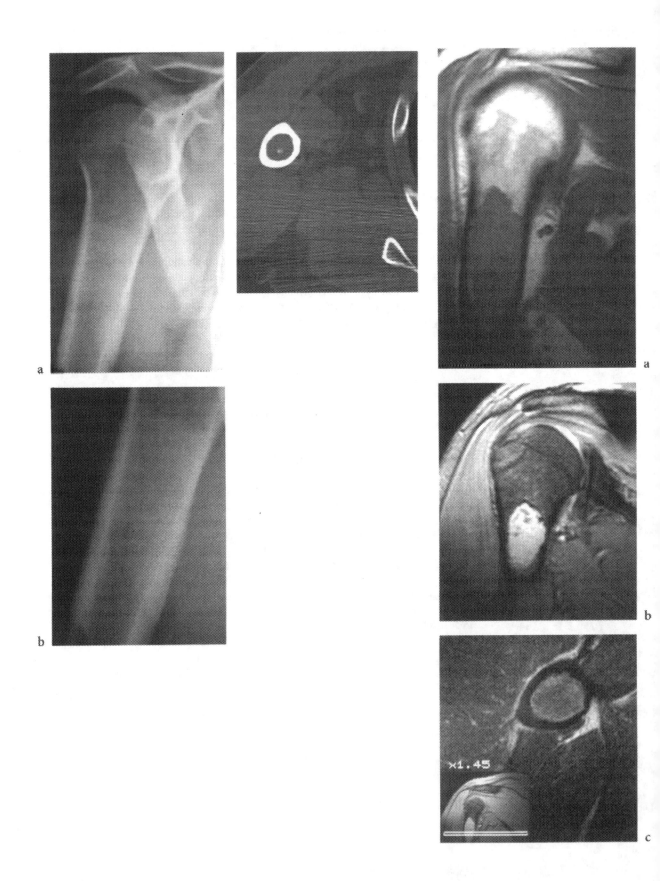

a

b

a

b

c

Why and What

1. Low-Grade Chondrosarcoma

The intramedullary high signal intensity on T2-weighted MRI indicates a chondromatous matrix of the lesion. The characteristic features pointing to low-grade chondrosarcoma are the size of the lesion (more than 4 cm), thickening of the cortex and tiny foci and septum-like enhancement within the lesion after administration of contrast medium. The sclerotic margin and the absence of periosteal reaction, soft tissue involvement, and of bone marrow edema are other features which are suggesting a low-grade chondrosarcoma.

2. Enchondroma

It is difficult to differentiate enchondroma from low-grade chondrosarcoma on the basis of signal intensity alone. However, the size of the lesion and the absence of significant central calcifications are in favor of low-grade chondrosarcoma. Additionally, the thickening of the cortex and the pattern of nodular and septum-like enhancement suggests low-grade chondrosarcoma. Enchondromas are common in the tubular bones of the hands and feet.

3. Fibrous Dysplasia

A slight ground-glass appearance of the lesion on the plain radiograph with minor calcifications on CT suggests a diagnosis of fibrous dysplasia; however, the signal intensity characteristics and the homogeneous appearance are more compatible with a chondromatous lesion.

4. Lymphoma

Lymphoma is much more common in the axial than the appendicular skeleton and particularly frequent in the vertebral bodies. There is also no calcified matrix, and on MRI homogeneous contrast enhancement would be expected.

5. Bone Infarction

Calcifications are typically more serpiginous or ring-like, not popcorn-like or amorphous, on plain films. On MRI only the acute phase of bone infarction demonstrates signal intensities similar to this case; however, the signal intensity on a T2-weighted sequence is less intense and a serpiginous morphology is expected. This is also true for chronic infarctions, which additionally show fatty tissue in the central portion of the lesion.

Final Diagnosis

Chondrosarcoma Grade 1

Definition. Chondrosarcoma which originates from the bone.

Incidence. Chrondrosarcoma is the fourth most common, after plasmocytoma, osteosarcoma, and Ewing sarcoma, among the primary tumors of the skeleton.

Age, sex distribution. Most grade 1 chondrosarcomas are found in the fourth, fifth and sixth decades. Males are more often affected than females.

Location. Central and metaphyseal areas of long bones; also seen in the pelvis and shoulder girdle.

Therapy. Radical intralesional excision or wide en bloc resection. Radiation and chemotherapy are effective only as palliative measures.

Prognosis. Chondrosarcomas are classified into grades 1–3:
grade 1 chondrosarcomas generally do not metastasize, although local recurrence after intralesional resection may occur; grade 2 chondrosarcomas are capable of metastasizing; grade 3 chondrosarcomas have a poor prognosis, even after oncologically adequate resection.

Case 17   Knee

History

This 27-year-old man had first noticed a mass in the right knee 3 years earlier. The mass had increased in size in the previous 6 months, and the patient suffered from moderate pain. He revealed no other clinical signs.

Imaging

1. Plain Film Radiographs

Fig. 17.1
Right knee, lateral
projection

Plain film radiographs reveal a soft tissue mass in the medio-dorsal aspect of the knee. Contact with the cortical bone of the femur can be suspected; however, there is no definite evidence of erosion or destruction of the cortical bone.

2. Magnetic Resonance Imaging

Fig. 17.2
Right knee

a T1-SE, sagittal plane
b T1-SE after contrast
administration, axial
plane
c T2-SE, fat saturation,
coronal plane

Magnetic resonance imaging reveals a large tumor in the anteromedial aspect of the right knee. The mass shows a diameter of approximately 10 × 3 × 3 cm. The tumor is hypointense and inhomogeneous with some septations on pre-contrast images and demonstrates inhomogeneous, bulky enhancement after administration of contrast medium (Figs. 17.2a, b). On pre- and postcontrast images the tumor is rather well circumscribed with smooth contours. On T2-weighted images there is no significant increase of signal intensity (Fig. 17.2c). Laterally and anteriorly the tumor has broad contact with the vastus intermedius and vastus medialis muscles, which are shifted anteriorly and laterally by the mass effect (Fig. 17.2b). A fat plane between the tumor and the muscle is not clearly visible, and infiltration must be suspected. Medially the tumor shows broad contact with the cortical bone of the femur, which appears thinned and irregular, but without definite evidence of invasion of the tumor into the bone marrow. The medial collateral ligament cannot be delineated and is probably infiltrated (Fig. 17.2c). On sagittal images, medially and ventrally infiltration of the joint must be suspected. There is also a second smaller, inhomogeneous but rather smoothly surrounded lesion laterally (ca. 4 × 1 cm) and a third lesion (2 × 1 cm) in the dorsal soft tissue compartments (Fig. 17.2b).

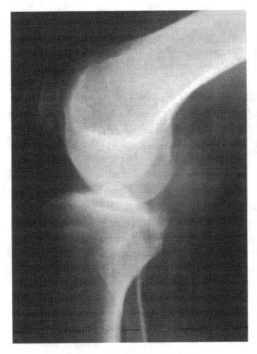

Fig. 17.1. Right knee, lateral projection

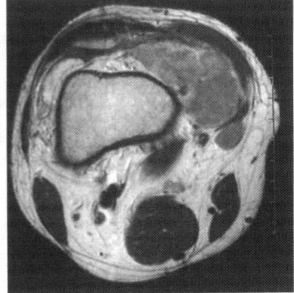

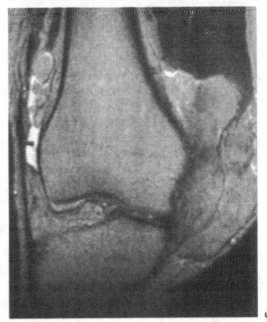

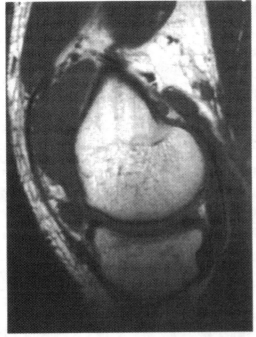

Fig. 17.2. Right knee

a T1-SE, sagittal plane
b T1-SE after contrast administration, axial plane
c T2-SE, fat saturation, coronal plane

Differential Diagnosis Based on Radiographs

– Soft tissue tumor

Differential Diagnosis Based on Radiographs and Further Studies

– Soft tissue tumor (malignant fibrous histiocytoma)
– Soft tissue tumor (fibrosarcoma, rhabdomyosarcoma)
– Metastases

Why and What

1. Plain film radiographs reveal a soft tissue mass but no more specific findings.
Malignant fibrous histiocytoma is the most common soft tissue tumor and demonstrates inhomogeneous hyperintense signal on T1 and T2 sequences.

2. Fibrosarcoma is a less frequent soft tissue tumor; however, theoretically its signal characteristics (homogeneous, intermediate to hypointense on T2-weighted images) would better resemble the pattern in our case.
Rhabdomyosarcoma is the second most frequent soft tissue tumor and is described to demonstrate mixed mild T2 hyperintensity.

3. Soft tissue metastases can demonstrate any signal intensity on T1- and T2-weighted images, depending on the fibrous and water content. The multiplicity of lesions in our case suggested this diagnosis, although soft tissue metastases are rare and the long clinical course would be atypical.

Final Diagnosis

Extraskeletal Ewing Sarcoma

Incidence. This tumor may occur as a primary soft tissue neoplasm without involvement of bone.
It mainly involves the soft tissue of the paravertebral region adjacent to the chest wall, the retroperitoneum, and the lower extremities. Distinction from other round-cell sarcomas is often difficult, and Ewing sarcoma is not always easy to distinguish microscopically from primitive forms of rhabdomyosarcoma, neuroblastoma, and neuroepithelioma.

Age, sex distribution. The tumor affects slightly more males than females and is seen in young adults between 15 and 30 years of age. The legs are rarely affected by extraskeletal Ewing sarcomas.

Clinical findings. Macroscopically, tumors are multilobulated and soft. Areas of colliquative necrosis and hemorrhage are frequently observed. Histologically, the aspect is the same as that of Ewing sarcoma of bone: uniform fields of small, round cells.

Therapy. Wide or radical resection in combination with chemotherapy or radiotherapy.

Prognosis. Reports are variable. In some series two-thirds of patients had a fatal outcome. Metastases are seen in the lung and the skeleton. Other authors report good results with intensive chemotherapy and radiation therapy in combination with local wide resection. Generally, the prognosis and treatment seems very similar to those for Ewing sarcoma of bone.

Remarks

Soft tissue tumors more than 3 cm in size must always be considered malignant, even with a rather smooth border. In this specific case major attention must be given to the possible intraarticular extension of the tumor and/or involvement of the collateral ligament which plays an important role for further therapy planning.

Case 18   Shoulder

History

This 53-year-old man presented with chronic pain in the left shoulder after an old subcapital fracture of the humerus. He had experienced several episodes of similar symptoms in previous years. On palpation he reported increased pain.

Imaging

1. Plain Film Radiographs

Fig. 18.1
Left shoulder,
a. p. projection

Plain film radiographs reveal evidence of an old subcapital fracture associated with reactive sclerosis and bone formation. In addition, however, the bone matrix in the area of the humeral head and the metaphysis shows an irregular pattern. The spongiotic bone is partly destroyed; there is an inhomogeneous pattern with radiolucent areas, predominantly subcortical, and areas of increased sclerosis. In the humeral head the cortical bone seems to have been destroyed.

No other lesions are evident. The surrounding soft tissue appears dense, with some shift of the fat line; however, no soft tissue calcifications are evident.

2. Magnetic Resonance Imaging

Fig. 18.2
Left shoulder

a T1-SE, axial plane
b T1-SE after contrast administration, axial plane
c T2-FSE, paracoronal plane

On T1-weighted images the fat marrow of the humeral head is altered to a great extent, demonstrating inhomogeneous, hypointense signal characteristics, predominantly in the dorsocranial aspect of the head, with only a small region of normal-appearing marrow (Fig. 18.2a). There is also evidence of a parosteal soft tissue component. Ventrally, and to a lesser extent dorsally, there are band-like hypointense soft tissue alterations, the fat planes are shifted or interrupted, and there are also small, round areas of homogeneous hypointense signal ventrally, with an diameter of 2.5 cm. After administration of contrast medium the affected areas demonstrate an enhancement which is particularly prominent in the parosteal soft tissue masses, predominantly adjacent to the ventral aspect of the humeral head (4×2 cm), and to a lesser extent dorsally (1×2 cm). Within these enhancing soft tissue masses, smaller areas remain hypointense and rather homogeneous. There is also significant enhancement of the synovia, which is thickened in parts and has a nodular appearance (Fig. 18.2b).

On T2-weighted images the osseous changes demonstrate an inhomogeneous character, with partly hyperintense and, partly hypointense signals. The adjacent soft tissue alterations are hyperintense, and the demarcated areas reveal a hyperintense homogeneous signal, indicating fluid-like collections adjacent to the anterior lateral aspect of the humeral head (maximum diameter: 2 cm). There is also an intraosseous fluid-like lesion in the subcortical aspect of the humeral head, and a small fluid collection dorsally, adjacent to the posterior glenoid (Fig. 18.2c).

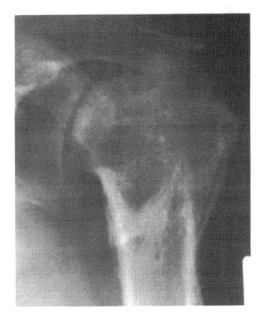

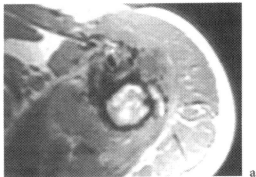

a

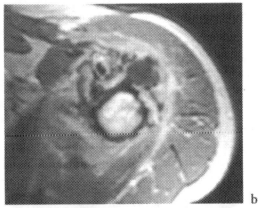

b

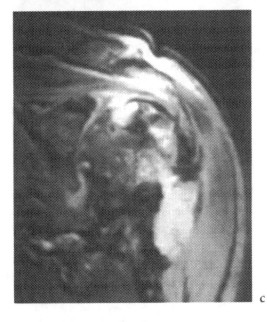

c

Why and What

1. MR imaging demonstrates prominent soft tissue involvement, with intra-osseous, articular and periarticular fluid collections, as well as evidence of synovitis. These signs indicate an inflammatory process or an associated inflammatory reaction.

2. There is evidence of an old fracture of the humerus together with osseous irregularities and spongiotic changes which indicate of a pathologic fracture. From plain film radiographs alone, therefore, a primary malignant bone lesion with a secondary pathological fracture is suspected. However the bone destruction with remodeling and sclerotic reaction points to a more chronic infiltrative process.

3. From plain film radiographs alone, basically a malignant lesion may be suspected as the underlying cause of the pathologic fracture. There is an irregular, partly destroyed pattern of the spongiotic bone and also signs of cortical destruction. However, the process appears more chronic and slowly progressing, as indicated by the reactive bone formation. Both metastases and plasmocytoma could reveal such patterns, and the age of the patient would also be consistent with these diagnoses.

4. MR imaging additionally reveals signs of a chronic inflammatory process, as demonstrated by the prominent soft tissue reaction adjacent to the lesion, evidence of a synovial reaction, and fluid collections. These findings are consistent with the course of chronic osteomyelitis, including osseous and soft tissue changes.

5. Even with the help of additional MR patterns, an underlying tumor cannot be excluded. Metastases could yield rather similar images. The associated signs of synovitis might be expected to be less prominent, but could potentially be present. Fluid collections in necrotic areas might also be present.

6. Another possibility involving an underlying inflammatory process is rapid destructive osteoarthritis which could potentially demonstrate similar patterns. However, the changes are found only within the humeral head, which makes this diagnosis unlikely, as we would expect similar changes also in the scapular component of the joint. The same considerations apply to rheumatoid arthritis.

Final Diagnosis

Inflammatory Postoperative Process (Chronic Osteomyelitis) with Reactive Spongiotic Proliferation

Definition. Osteomyelitis implies an infection of bone and bone marrow. The routes of contamination can be hematogenous, spread of a contiguous infection, direct implantation, and postoperative infection. Postoperative infections may occur by contamination from adjacent tissue, by hematogenous spread, or by inoculation. The most common pathogen is *Staphylococcus aureus*.

Incidence. 1 – 2 % after surgery.

Age, sex distribution. There is no significant relation to age or gender.

Therapy. Surgical debridement and excision of all bone necrosis and the adjacent scar formation and long-term administration of antibiotics.

Prognosis. Chronic osteomyelitis can recur at any time, particularly with deficiencies of the immune system. Nevertheless, adequate surgical treatment significantly decreases the chance of recurrence.

Case 19   Shoulder

History

This 10-year-old girl presented with a history of pain and swelling in the right shoulder for 9 months. The pain increased with palpation, but no other symptoms or skin changes were evident.

Imaging

1. Plain Film Radiographs

Fig. 19.1
Right scapula,
a. p. projection

Plain film radiographs reveal a huge radiolucent lesion in the right acromion and the adjacent lateral and superior aspect of the scapula. The lesion is markedly expansive, with thinning and prominent displacement of the cortical bone. However, there is no evidence of destruction. There is loss of the regular spongious pattern, and the matrix shows a rather homogeneous character without evidence of calcifications or reactive or new bone formation. However, septations within the lesion are clearly delineated. No further lesions are evident, and the soft tissue is normal.

2. Computed Tomography

Fig. 19.2
Right scapula, axial
plane, bone window

Computed tomography reveals that the lesion is located mainly in the acromion and demonstrates its marked expansive character. Using a bone algorithm the cortical bone can be clearly identified, and it is thinned and displaced anteriorly and posteriorly. In the dorsal aspect of the acromion there is even evidence of loss of cortical bone, as it cannot be visualized continuously. There are multiple bony septations within the lesion which demonstrates a thinned and irregular surface. The lesion measures approximately 5 × 8 cm in the transverse plane. A smaller lesion with similar characteristics can be seen in the adjacent aspect of the scapula (4 × 2.5 cm). Using a soft tissue algorithm, in both lesions an area of intermediate signal intensity can be delineated in the dependent aspect, with a fluid-like density (28.3 Hounsfield units) below a horizontal level and a low signal intensity area above. This represents a fluid level.

3. Magnetic Resonance Imaging

Fig. 19.3
Right scapula

a T1-SE after contrast
administration, coronal
plane
b T1-SE after contrast
administration with fat
saturation (STIR), axial
plane
c T2-weighted image
with fat saturation
(STIR), axial plane

Magnetic resonance imaging underlines the observations from the CT images, but demonstrates even more clearly the different tissue qualities. On T1-weighted images the lesions show a multilobulated expansive character with hypointense signal characteristics (Fig. 19.3a). After administration of contrast medium, there is marked marginal enhancement, whereas the central parts remain unenhanced. Contrast-enhanced, fat-suppressed T1-weighted images also clearly demonstrate the fluid levels (Fig. 19.3b). T2-weighted and STIR images show high signal isointense with fluid, with evidence of fluid-fluid levels with lower signal intensity of the dependent portion and higher signal intensity above (Fig. 19.3c).
There is no periosseous soft tissue reaction.

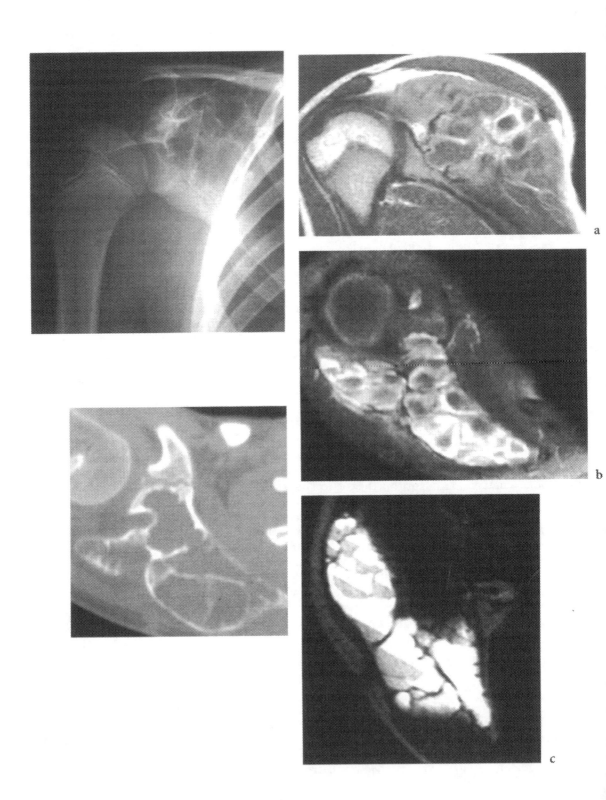

a

b

c

Differential Diagnosis Based on Radiographs

– Aneurysmal bone cyst

Differential Diagnosis Based on Radiographs and Further Studies

– Aneurysmal bone cyst

Why and What

Aneurysmal Bone Cyst

There is an expansive multicystic lesion in the right acromion and scapula of a 10-years-old girl. Although the matrix of the lesion cannot be further specified on plain film radiographs, the diagnosis of aneurysmal bone cyst is highly suspected. CT and MRI clearly demonstrate the fluid-fluid levels.

The findings on MRI are characteristic. Internal septations, cystic lobulations, and fluid-fluid levels of various signal intensities are obvious. An expanded low-signal-intensity rim surrounding the lesion can be seen. Portions of the lesion have high signal intensity on T1-weighted and T2-weighted images. Fluid-fluid levels may also be seen in teleangiectatic osteosarcoma, giant cell tumor, cystic chondroblastoma, and tumoral calcinosis.

The multicystic appearance of the lesion in the case with its expansive character and the evidence of the fluid-fluid levels is almost pathognomonic.

Final Diagnosis

Aneurysmal Bone Cyst

Definition. An aneurysmal bone cyst is a pseudotumoral lesion of bone. It may arise de novo in bone where a definite preexisting lesion cannot be demonstrated in the tissue. On the other hand areas similar to an aneurysmal bone cyst can be found in various benign conditions and even, occasionally, in malignant tumors. The cause of the lesion is unknown.

Incidence. Aneurysmal bone cyst occurs infrequently. Generally it is half as frequent as giant-cell tumor.

Age, sex distribution. There is a slight predilection for females, with a male to female ratio of 0.8:1. Aneurysmal bone cyst occurs predominantly between the ages of 10 and 20 years (70%), although it is observed at any age.

Location. Aneurysmal bone cysts are found in all parts of the skeleton. The regions mainly affected are the knee and proximal femur and the vertebral column. In the vertebral column, aneurysmal bone cyst tends to involve the posterior elements.

Therapy. Intralesional resection of the aneurysmal bone cyst associated with the use of local adjuvants (phenol, liquid nitrogen, cement) and bone grafting is the most common treatment modality. In favorable sites, segmental resections (ribs) are performed. In unfavorable sites, such as the vertebral column and the pelvis, selective arterial embolization, single or repeated, is often successful.

Prognosis. The prognosis is excellent. An aneurysmal bone cyst nearly always heals. The recurrence rate after incomplete curettage is 10–15%.

Remarks

Aneurysmal bone cyst is a lesion characterized by a highly expansive appearance. There are two types:

- A primary cyst without an associated lesion
- A secondary cyst that occurs in association with a bone tumor

Potential tumors associated with a secondary bone cyst are:

- Giant cell tumor
- Osteosarcoma
- Solitary bone cyst
- Nonossifying fibroma
- Fibrous dysplasia
- Metastatic carcinoma
- Chondromyxoid fibroma
- Hemangioendothelioma
- Osteoblastoma
- Chondroblastoma
- Fibromyxohemangioma

A nontumorous cause of secondary bone cyst is fracture.

Case 20   Knee

History

This 56-year-old woman complained of stress-dependent pain of the right knee joint in the area of the lateral condyles extending distally to the middle third of the lower leg. Pain had started after a trauma two years earlier. The patient underwent arthroscopic meniscectomy; however, the symptoms were not relieved.

Imaging

1. Conventional Tomography

Fig. 20.1
Right knee,
a. p. projection

Conventional tomography of the right knee reveals an osteolytic lesion in an epiphyseal subchondral location in the lateral femoral condyle. The lateral margin of the lesion is well defined with a subtle sclerotic rim; the medial border is not well delineated (Fig. 20.1).

2. Computed Tomography

Fig. 20.2
Right knee, axial plane,
bone window

Computed tomography reveals an osteolytic lesion in the medial dorsal aspect of the lateral condyle with a sclerotic rim laterally. There is no definite border medially, where this process is opened towards the adjacent soft tissue. The lesion has an erosive character and in its proximal aspect also reveals subtle calcifications. The diameter of the lesion is 1 cm (Fig. 20.2).

3. Magnetic Resonance Imaging

Fig. 20.3
Right knee

a T1-SE, sagittal plane
b T2-weighted image,
sagittal plane

T1-weighted SE images reveal the lesion with hypointense signal in the dorsal aspect of the lateral femoral condyle (Fig. 20.3a). On T2-weighted images the lesion shows centrally inhomogeneous high signal and low signal peripherally (Fig. 20.3b). There is some evidence of intraosseous and extraosseous components of the lesion, as a part of the lesion extends beyond the osseous margin. Medially and ventrally, at the border to the bone there is low signal intensity on T1- and T2-weighted images. No signal changes are evident within the bone marrow.
There are also signal alterations within Hoffa's fat pad and in the area of the medial meniscus, consistent with postoperative changes after meniscectomy. There are extensive degenerative changes in the lateral meniscus and an osteochondral defect in the lateral tibial and femoral plateau.

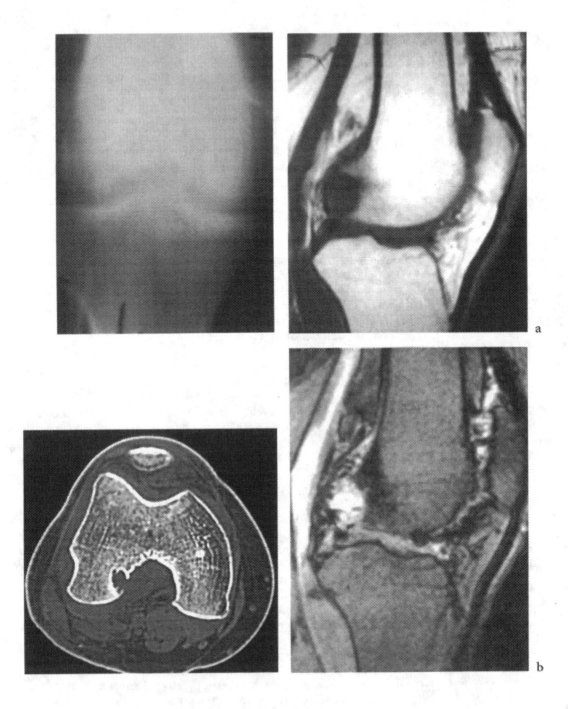

a

b

Why and What

1. Intraosseous Ganglion

Besides the postoperative findings, the extensive degenerative changes of the remaining meniscus and the osteochondral defects in the medial area of the joint, there is evidence of an osteolytic lesion in the mediodorsal aspect of the lateral femoral condyle. It is an erosive, bony lesion with sclerotic margins indicating slow growth and a reactive reparative process. The mass itself is inhomogeneous, with intra- and extraosseous parts. The lesion therefore is not necessarily a primarily bony lesion; a soft tissue lesion with bone invasion is possible.

The location and the formation of the lesion would be consistent with an intraosseous ganglion, slowly eroding the cortical bone. However, the signal characteristics are rather inhomogeneous, with hypointensity on both T1- and T2-weighted images and only centrally hyperintense signal on T2-SE images.

2. Meniscal Cyst

The location and the type of bony reaction could also be compatible with a meniscal cyst; moreover, the lesion shows contact with the lateral meniscus. Nevertheless, we would expect a more homogeneous appearance and higher signal intensities on both T1- and T2-weighted images.

3. Chondroblastoma

The signal characteristics demonstrate an inhomogeneous mass of popcorn appearance, which could resemble a chondroblastoma, with reactive sclerosis of the adjacent bone lesions. However, there is no perifocal bone marrow edema and no soft tissue mass, which tends to rule out this diagnosis.

4. Cystic Lesion, Giant-Cell Tumor

Given the location and appearance, a cystic lesion, an aneurysmal bone cyst or a giant-cell tumor could be concluded from plain film radiographs alone; however, these diagnoses can be excluded by MRI.

Final Diagnosis

Intraosseous Ganglion

Definition. The intraosseus ganglion develops within the bone in the proximity of a joint. The differential diagnosis includes cyst associated with degenerative joint disease. The anatomo-pathological nature of these cysts is the same as that of the more wellknown and common ganglions of the soft tissue.

Synonyms. Ganglion of bone, subchondral bone cyst, juxtaarticular bone cyst, synovial cyst of bone.

Incidence. Intraosseous ganglions are seen occasionally.

Age, sex distribution. The lesion is observed in adult hond.
There is a predilection for males, with a sex ratio of 1.5:1.

Location. The ankle, the knee, the hip region, and the wrist are mainly affected. Generally the ganglion is located in the vicinity of a joint surface.

Therapy. Intralesional resection and packing of the cavity with bone chips.

Prognosis. In exceptional cases there may be a recurrence, even when the excision was complete, due to mucoid transformation of the surrounding connective tissue.

Remarks

The classic appearance of a ganglion is hypo- to hyperintense signal on T1-weighted images and hyperintense signal on T2-weighted images. In this particular case, the hypointense signals on T1-weighted images and only central hyperintense signal on T2-weighted images indicate a rather fibrous matrix with only of little water content. Such changes might appear over a long course of disease.

Case 21   Foot

History

This 46-year-old man presented with a swelling and pain in the medial and lateral aspect of the right hindfoot. On clinical evaluation a rather firm mass could be palpated; there were no skin alterations and no evidence of other symptoms or lesions.

Imaging

1. Plain Film Radiographs

Fig. 21.1

a Right foot, lateral projection
b Left foot, lateral projection

Plain film radiographs reveal a smoothly contoured enlargement of the sinus tarsi (Fig. 21.1). Particularly concerning the cranial aspect of the calcaneus a prominent concavity is obvious. There is evidence of some cortical reaction; however, there are no signs of osseous erosion. The bony matrix in the area of the lesion demonstrates increased radiolucency, but the spongious structure appears regular. There is no evidence of associated soft tissue involvement, and there are no calcifications or ossifications. Otherwise there is a small cystic lesion in the calcaneus and mild degenerative changes.

2. Magnetic Resonance Imaging

Fig. 21.2

a Both ankles, T1-SE, coronal plane
b Both ankles, T1-SE after contrast administration, coronal plane
c Right foot, sinus tarsi, T2-SE with fat suppression (STIR), coronal plane

T1-weighted images reveal a hypointense lesion in the medial caudal aspect of the talus, expanding into the sinus tarsi and infiltrating the superior lateral aspect of the calcaneus with a transverse diameter of 2.5 × 2.5 cm and a craniocaudal extension of 4 cm. Within the sinus tarsi it follows the intertarsal ligaments, and the ligaments of the tarsal sinus cannot be delineated (Fig. 21.2a). After administration of contrast medium the lesion shows only moderate enhancement (Fig. 21.2b). On T2-weighted images the mass remains centrally hypointense and inhomogeneous, with only a slight increase of signal intensity in the peripheral parts of the lesion. On fat-suppressed (STIR) images the lesion demonstrates various degrees of high signal intensities, with centrally only small, almost punctate areas of low signal (Fig. 21.2c). The lesion has a lobulated character with smooth borders. An intraosseous expansion is visible; however, the corresponding borders of the adjacent bony components are also rather smooth with a concave contour and no or only a minimal reaction of the perifocal bone marrow.

There is a prominent soft tissue reaction with edema and swelling extending laterally more than medially. There is also a small fluid collection within the joint space.

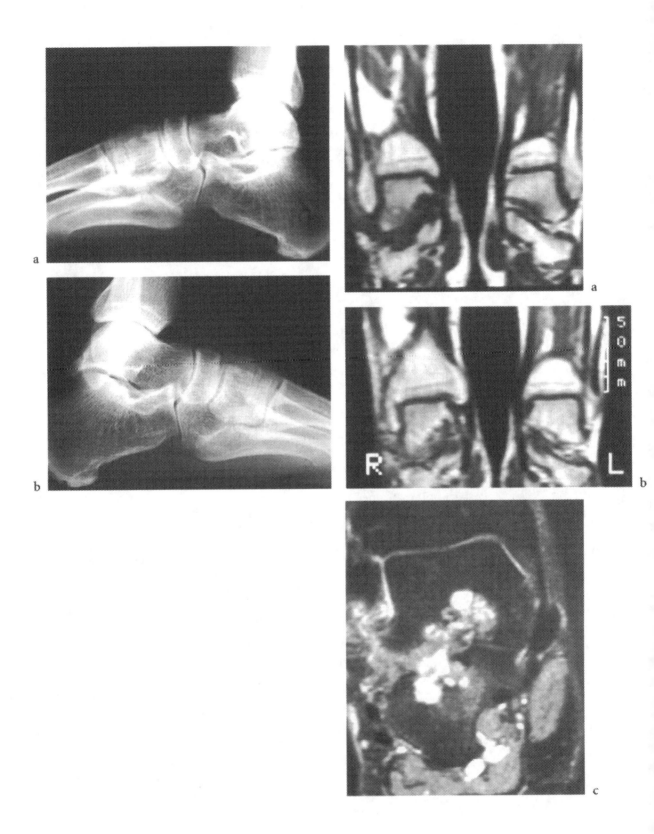

Why and What

1. Giant-Cell Tumor of the Tendon Sheath/Pigmented Villonodular Synovitis

There is evidence of a mass arising maximum in the sinus tarsi, expanding into the adjacent bones. The smooth concave contours of the bony lesion with some sclerotic reaction, the near-absence of bone marrow edema, and the moderate enhancement indicate a rather slowly growing process. The appearance of the mass indicates a primarily extraosseous lesion with slow intraosseous expansion. As there are no typical signs of chondromatous origin, one has to suspect that the lesion arose from intraarticular soft tissue elements. As the signal characteristics are compatible with a partly fibrous and partly lobular cyst-like structure, the diagnosis of a giant-cell tumor of the tendon sheath, arising from chronic proliferations, appears possible. Further foci of hemosiderin deposition can be suspected as punctate lesions without signal on all pulse sequences. The mass itself also might not increase in signal intensity on T2-weighted images because of its hemosiderin content. The location and the age of the patient are also consistent with giant-cell tumor. Although histologically both tumors arise from the same matrix, pigmented villonodular synovitis (PVNS) usually shows more aggressive characteristics with more prominent erosion of the adjacent bone. Therefore, benign giant-cell tumor of the tendon sheath is the first choice in this case.

2. Extraosseous Ganglion with Intraosseous Expansion

The multicystic appearance with the smooth erosion of the bone might also be consistent with an intraosseously expanding ganglion. However, the low signal characteristics on T1- and T2-weighted images are rather atypical and could only be explained by a low protein content.

3. Chondroma

On the basis of STIR images alone, the lobulated, hyperintense signal characteristics of the lesion with a somewhat cloudy appearance could be consistent with a slowly growing chondromatous lesion. However, the low signal on T2-SE images would be rather atypical. Moreover, although they are not mandatory, there are none of the cloud- or popcorn-like calcifications evident on plain film radiographs.

Final Diagnosis

Giant-Cell Tumor of the Tendon Sheath/Pigmented Villonodular Synovitis

Definition. Hyperplastic production of synovial tissue of joints, tendon sheaths, bursae or fibrous tissue adjacent to the tendons. PVNS may be present in two manifestations:

- Diffuse villonodular form
- Localized nodular form

Synonyms. Xanthoma, xanthogranuloma, benign synovialoma, giant-cell tumor of the tendon sheath, fibrous histiocytoma of the synovium.

Incidence. The paratendineous nodular synovitis is particularly frequent in the hand. Joint affections are relatively rare.

Age, sex distribution. The highest incidence is between 20 and 40 years of age, but the range is 10–75 years. There is no gender predilection.

Location. PVNS is frequently observed in the fingers, where it occurs in the sheath of the flexor tendons. It is not very common in the foot in relation to the flexor and extensor tendons. Of the joints, more than 75% of all cases occur in the knee, followed by the hip, wrist, ankle, and shoulder.

Therapy. In the localized nodular form marginal excision is easy and, if it is completely performed, there is no recurrence. In the diffuse villonodular form, complete surgical excision may be difficult or impossible. There is a high risk of local recurrence.

Remarks

Radiographically, due to the smooth contours and the rather regular bone structure, the lesion within the sinus tarsi can easily be missed. Comparison of left and right definitely helps to detect the lesion.

PVNS and villonodular tenosynovitis are chronic proliferations, probably caused by inflammatory reactions that occur in the synovia of the joints, tendons, and bursae. PVNS is classified as a diffuse form that affects the entire synovial membrane and as a localized form that affects tendon sheaths or a small part of the synovium. The cyst-like defects have sharp and sclerotic margins, which rarely may progress to joint destruction. MRI is of great help in characterizing the lesion due to the possibility of subtle detection of blood products (hemosiderin), characteristic for this lesion. Hemosiderin shows low signal intensity on all sequences, which is otherwise only seen with calcifications. With the combined reading of plain film radiographs, the differentiation is easy. Also the low signal on T2-weighted images, rather atypical for blastomatous lesions, is due to a diffuse amount of hemosiderin within the lesion.

Case 22   Knee

History

This 42-year-old woman observed a swelling in the left knee with increasing pain over the previous 3 years. The patient underwent conservative and local injection therapy, with no relief of pain. On clinical examination a rather firm mass was palpated at an infrapatellar location. No other clinical signs were evident. Blood count was normal.

Imaging

1. Plain Film Radiographs

Fig. 22.1
Left knee, lateral projection

Radiographs reveal a soft tissue density in the left knee ventrally centered below the patella and at the level of the knee joint. In the lateral projection, bizarre streaky and globular irregular calcifications can be observed. The adjacent cortical bone of the femur, the tibia and patella in this area are normal; there is no evidence of an associated osseous lesion. There is subtle evidence of chondrocalcinosis of the medial meniscus (Fig. 22.1).

2. Magnetic Resonance Imaging

Fig. 22.2
Left knee

a T1-SE, sagittal plane
b T2-weighted image, sagittal plane
c STIR, coronal plane

T1-weighted images demonstrate complete obliteration of the normally hyperintense signal intensity of Hoffa's fat pad, which is diffusely hypointense in this case, associated with small central areas of complete signal loss (Fig. 22.2a). On T2-weighted images the lesion shows a pseudocystic appearance, with multiple, well-circumscribed round or ovoid formations, up to 8 mm in size, with high, fluid-like signal intensities within Hoffa's fat pad. These lesions are seperated by septation-like bands of lower signal intensities (Fig. 22.2b). The lesion expands intraarticularly and at the level of the cruciate ligaments extends dorsally into the joint, where it reaches the anterior surface of the anterior cruciate ligament. The anterior medial meniscus cannot be defined regularly. The lesion further demonstrates in its posterior extension broad contact with the ventral aspect of the medial femoral condyle, proximally the patellar apex, ventrally the patellar ligament, and distally the anterior surface of the tibial plateau. These contact surfaces are smooth, and there is no evidence of infiltration of these adjacent structures. There is also no associated marrow edema or any other reaction in the adjacent bone.

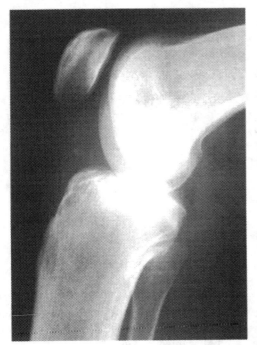

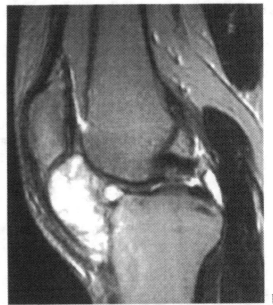

b

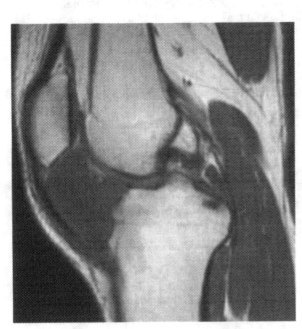

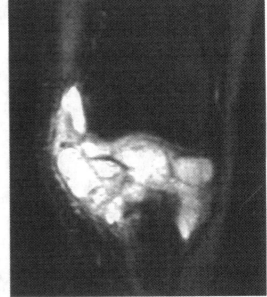

c

Why and What

There is a slowly growing mass in the anterior soft tissue compartment of the knee with complete obliteration and transformation of Hoffa's fat pad and with clearly visible extension into the joint space. The lesion shows signal characteristics resembling fluid with a multicystic appearance, and the lesion can be considered primarily extraosseous. Calcifications, evident on the plain film radiographs, may be primarily related to the lesion, but could also be due to the injection therapy.

1. Chondromatosis

Plain film radiographs provide evidence of a soft tissue tumor, owing to the absence of erosion or destruction of the adjacent bones. However, further specification is difficult. The observed calcifications are rather bizarre and not in a typically could-like formation, but could be consistent with a chondromatous matrix of the tumor. Nevertheless, almost any mesenchymal soft tissue tumor can demonstrate calcifications. Moreover, the calcifications are not unequivocally distinguishable from reactive calcifications owing to the injection therapy.

2. Lipomatous Tumor

As the lesion arises from Hoffa's fat pad, an atypical lipoma or liposarcoma has to be considered. The matrix of lipomatous tumors can vary depending on the amount of pluripotent and/or fat cells, and can therefore resemble a diverse spectrum of matrix signals, although the obviously complete loss of fat tissue (T1-SE sequences) would be rather atypical.

3. Soft Tissue Tumor

Any other soft tissue tumor arising from pluripotent mesenchymal cells can produce a variety of signal characteristics, from fluid-like to solid.

4. Synovial Tumor

The location is compatible with a synovial tumor, and a synovialoma theoretically could demonstrate signal characteristics basically similar to those seen in this case. The bizarre calcifications and the age of the patient would also be consistent with this diagnosis. However, synovialomas are highly malignant fibroblastic tumors, highly vascularized and associated with bony erosions, not visible in this patient. Also, fluid-fluid levels, as might appear in a synovialoma, are not evident. Pigmented villonodular synovitis is associated with osseous lesions and features blood products, neither of which are not evident in our case, and can therefore be excluded.

Final Diagnosis

Articular Chondromatosis and Meniscal Chondromatosis

Definition. This lesion is a new formation of well-differentiated hyaline cartilage within the joint synovial membrane, the tendon sheath or the bursal
mucosa.

Incidence. Relatively rare.

Age, sex distribution. Observed in adulthood, frequently between 30 and 50
years of age. Predilection for males.

Location. Fifty percent of all cases are localized in the knee, followed by the
elbow and other large joints (shoulder, wrist, hip, ankle). The extraarticular
form is observed in most cases in the fingers, more rarely in the hand, wrist,
foot, and ankle, and is nearly always related to a tendon.

Symptoms. Symptoms generally progress very slowly. A few years elapse between first symptoms and treatment. Typically, the symptoms are pain,
limited joint motion, joint crackling, blocking, and synovial effusion, and
loose bodies are palpated.

Therapy. Synovectomy, which should be as complete as possible, and removal
of loose bodies. In paratendinous forms the treatment of choice is simple
marginal excision of the nodule.

Prognosis. The course is protracted. After synovectomy, even if only partial,
recurrences are infrequent.

Case 23   Shoulder

History

This 46-year-old man had already undergone surgery for a chondrosarcoma (grade 2–3) in the acromioclavicular joint 18 months previously. He suffered from continuous pain and soft tissue swelling.

Imaging

1. Plain Film Radiographs

Fig. 23.1
Right shoulder, axial plane

Plain film radiographs demonstrate the postoperative status in the area of the acromioclavicular and glenohumeral joints, with the resection of the distal part of the clavicle and the acromion. The osseous borders are well delineated, with only some slight irregularity which might be due to reactive changes. Some soft tissue swelling might be suspected, but these is no evidence of a mass. There is only a vague reduction of the regular trabecular pattern in the humeral head, without evidence of lytic changes (Fig. 23.1).

2. Magnetic Resonance Imaging

Fig. 23.2
Right shoulder

a T1-SE, axial plane
b T2-weighted image with fat suppression (STIR), coronal plane
c T1-SE after contrast administration with fat suppression (SPIR), coronal plane
d T1-SE after contrast administration with fat suppression (SPIR), axial plane

Magnetic resonance imaging reveals a mass in the operated area of the previous acromioclavicular joint. The mass extends dorsally and inferiorly with broad contact to the posterolateral aspect of the humeral head. There is also a smaller part extending into the humeral head. The osseous defect shows diameter of 1.5×1.5 cm.
The mass has a diameter of 5×6 cm in axial planes and a craniocaudal extension of 7 cm. Signal is low and inhomogeneous on T1-SE images (Fig. 23.2a). On STIR images (Fig. 23.2b) the lesion is hyperintense and demonstrates multiple septations. The mass is well circumscribed and shows mass effect on surrounding structures; however, there is no infiltration of surrounding soft tissue structures. After administration of contrast medium, strong enhancement of the irregular, thickened and nodular margins can be observed (Figs. 23.2c, d). The matrix of the lesion remains partly unenhanced and hypointense, indicating larger areas of cystic parts, together with an extensively enhancing irregular and cloudy appearance of other parts.

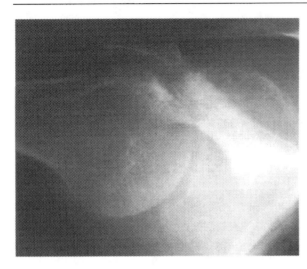

Fig. 23.1. Right shoulder, axial plane
◄

Fig. 23.2. Right shoulder

a T1-SE, axial plane
b T2-weighted image with fat suppression (STIR), coronal plane
c T1-SE after contrast administration with fat suppression (SPIR), coronal plane
d T1-SE after contrast administration with fat suppression (SPIR), axial plane
▼

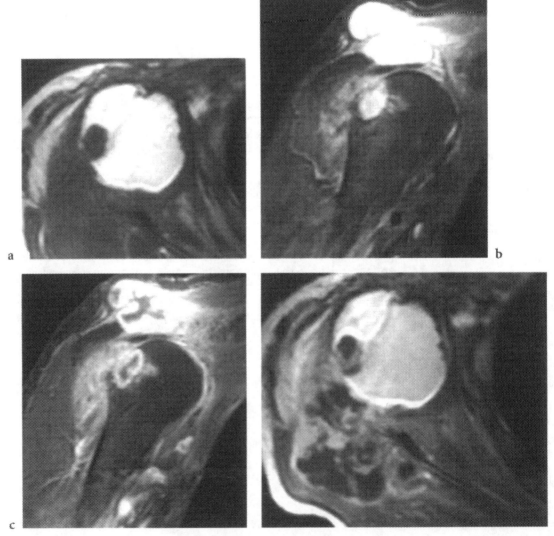

Differential Diagnosis Based on Radiographs

– Postoperative changes
– Recurrence
– Inflammation

Differential Diagnosis Based on Radiographs and Further Studies

– Recurrence

Why and What

1. Recurrence

This is an inhomogeneous, partly cystic, partly solid mass arising in the area of previous surgery. It has broad contact with and partly invades the humeral head. The matrix is hyperintense on T2-weighted images, and the lesion shows extensive enhancement and irregular walls. All these findings strongly suggest a tumor recurrence with partly necrotic transformation.

2. Extensive Inflammatory Changes

Theoretically the signal characteristics could be those of an inflammatory process. Enhancement of thickened irregular margins can be observed, together with a partly cystic, partly solid appearance in patients with rheumatoid arthritis or an otherwise aggressive inflammatory disease. However, invasion of bone indicates a very aggressive character or a late stage of disease, and the patient does not show the clinical signs of inflammatory disease.

3. Postoperative Changes

This diagnosis is very unlikely. Although the lesion shows partly cystic areas which might be consistent with postoperative changes, the extensive enhancement, the amount of solid components, the extension of the lesion with its invasion of bone, and the irregularity of the borders are not consistent with postoperative changes such as scar tissue, granulation tissue, or seroma.

Final Diagnosis

Recurrence of Chondrosarcoma

Definition. Chondrosarcoma which originates from inside the bone.

Synonyms. Central chondrosarcoma.

Incidence. Among the primary tumors of the skeleton chondrosarcoma is the fourth most common after plasmocytoma, osteosarcoma, and Ewing sarcoma.

Age, sex distribution. Chondrosarcomas are most common in the fourth, fifth, and sixth decades of life. Males are more frequently affected than females.

Location. Central, metaphyseal ends of long bones; also seen in pelvis and shoulder girdle.

Therapy. Radical excision or limb salvage en bloc. Radiation therapy and chemotherapy are effective only as palliative measures.

Prognosis. Chondrosarcomas are classified into grades 1–3: grade 1 chondrosarcomas generally do not metastasize, although local recurrence after intralesional resection may occur; grade 2 chondrosarcomas are capable of metastasizing; grade 3 chondrosarcomas have a poor prognosis, even after oncologically adequate resection.

Remarks

Postoperative changes are difficult to distinguish from tumor recurrence, especially in early follow-up investigations, and often can only be revealed in the course of repeated ongoing follow-up. Enhancement is also evident in postoperative changes, but should decrease with time, as should the perifocal edema. Irregular, thickened walls and particularly loss of decreased enhancement or even increased enhancement in follow-up investigations should always arouse strong suspicion of tumor recurrence.

Case 24   Distal Femur, Knee

History

This 12-year-old boy suffered acute onset of pain following a minor trauma in the right distal femur.

Imaging

1. Plain Film Radiographs

Fig. 24.1
Right distal femur
and knee joint, lateral
projection

X-rays reveal a well-defined ovoid radiolucency in the metadiaphyseal area of the right distal femur. The lesion measures 4 × 2.5 cm. The center of the lesion is located posteriomedially. The lesion has an mildly expansive character, with bowing of the medial and dorsal contour of the femur. The cortical bone of this area is thin and in one place cannot be delineated at all. The matrix of the lesion is rather homogeneous; the border is well defined. There is a fracture line arising from the anterior aspect of the femur extending through the lucency posteriorly and involving the cortical bone posteriorly, where a subtle step in the cortical contour is evident (Fig. 24.1). There is moderate soft tissue swelling around the lesion.

2. Magnetic Resonance Imaging

Fig. 24.2
Right distal femur

a T2-weighted image
with fat suppression
(STIR), sagittal plane
b T2-weighted image,
axial plane
c T1-SE, sagittal plane

Magnetic resonance imaging demonstrates the lesion as an area of high signal intensity on STIR and T2-weighted lesions (Figs. 24.2 a, b). The lesion is well demarcated and has broad contact with the posteriomedial aspect of the cortical bone, which is thin. A striking feature is the presence of different intensities of high signal within the lesion, sharply linearly demarcated and shift depending on the body position on axial and sagittal images, indicating fluid-fluid levels (Fig. 24.2 b). There is also a subtle septation going vertically through the anterior aspect of the lesion, and a more irregular, hypointense, partly linear, partly streaky area (ca. 1 cm) is visible in the dorsobasal part of the lesion.

On STIR images an irregular hyperintense line arises from the anterior aspect of the lesion, expanding ventrally to the cortical bone. On T1-weighted images the lesion shows homogeneously low signal intensity and the irregular ventrally expanding line is also hypointense (Fig. 24.2 c). There is a poorly defined area of high signal intensity within the bone marrow proximally and, less prominent, distally of the lesion.

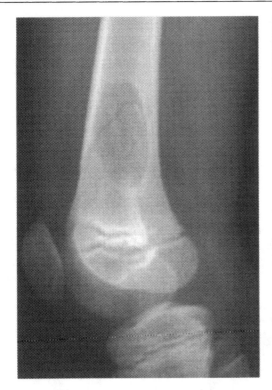

Fig. 24.1. Right distal femur and knee joint, lateral projection

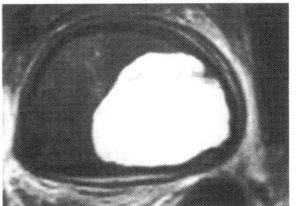

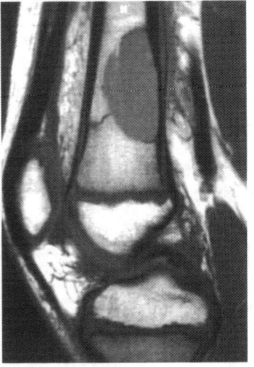

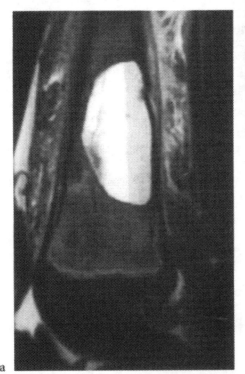

Fig. 24.2. Right distal femur

a T2-weighted image with fat suppression (STIR), sagittal plane
b T2-weighted image, axial plane
c T1-SE, sagittal plane

Why and What

1. Aneurysmatic Bone Cyst with Secondary Pathologic Fracture

The lesion has a typical appearance, featuring a radiolucency of the central axis with slight ballooning of a thinned cortex. The aneurysmal bony effect is not very obvious in this case. The long axis of the lesion is parallel to the long axis of the bone, and there is very subtle periosteal new bone formation or reactive bone formation at the posterior margin, perhaps owing to previous trauma. The character of the lesion and its metadiaphyseal location suggest the diagnosis of an aneurysmal bone cyst, although a malignant bone tumor cannot be excluded by plain radiographs alone.

The MRI findings are very characteristic, and the fluid-fluid levels almost pathognomonic. They might appear, however, with tumor necrosis or in teleangiectatic osteosarcoma. There is also evidence of some smaller amounts of blood products. The perifocal diffuse bone marrow edema is supposedly due to the recent trauma, and the fracture line is also clearly visible as an irregular hyperintense line on T2- and a hypointense line on T1-weighted images. Owing to the homogeneous signal characteristics of the lesion an underlying tumor can be ruled out. The acute posttraumatic onset of pain leads us to suspect a pathologic fracture after minimal trauma at the site of a preexisting lesion.

2. Nonossifying Fibroma with Secondary Pathologic Fracture

Nonossifying fibroma is characteristically seen in the metaphysis of long bones, has an off-axis appearance, manifests as an ovoid radiolucency, the peak incidence is in the second decade of life, and pathologic fractures may occur. The margins, however, are usually scallopped, with the inner margin having a sclerotic appearance, which is not the case here.

3. Aneurysmatic Bone Cyst with Underlying Bone Lesion and Secondary Pathologic Fracture

The matrix of the lesion is not as homogeneous as might be expected with a primary aneurysmal bone cyst. A secondary aneurysmal bone cyst can occur in association with a bone tumor. Lesions that theoretically could be present on the basis of the MRI findings in this case are fibrous dysplasia and chondromyxoid fibroma. An osteosarcoma can also be associated with an aneurysmal bone cyst; however, the MRI appearance is not that of osteosarcoma in this case.

Final Diagnosis

Aneurysmal Bone Cysts

Definition. Aneurysmal bone cyst is a pseudotumoral lesion. It may arise de novo in bone where a definite preexisting lesion cannot be demonstrated. On the other hand, areas similar to an aneurysmal bone cyst can be found in various benign conditions and even, occasionally, in malignant tumors. The cause of the lesion is unknown.

Incidence. Aneurysmal bone cysts occur infrequently. Generally they are half as common as giant-cell tumor.

Age, sex distribution. Aneurysmal bone cysts occur predominantly (70%) between the ages of 10 and 20 years, although they can be observed at any age. There is a slight predilection for females, with a male to female ratio of 0.8:1.

Location. Aneurysmal bone cysts are found in all parts of the skeleton. The region around the knee, the proximal femur, and the vertebral column are mainly affected. In the vertebral column aneurysmal bone cysts tend to involve the posterior elements.

Therapy. Intralesional resection of the aneurysmal bone cyst associated with the use of local adjuvants (phenol, liquid nitrogen, cement) and bone grafting is the most common treatment modality. In favorable sites, segmental resections (ribs) are performed. In unfavorable sites such as the vertebral column and the pelvis, selective arterial embolization, single or repeated, is often successful.

Prognosis. The prognosis is excellent. An aneurysmal bone cyst nearly always heals. The recurrence rate after incomplete curettage is 10%–15%.

Remarks

The fluid-fluid level as depicted on MRI is pathognomonic. It is due to sedimentation of different protein concentrations within the lesion. Moreover, the location of the lesion and the age of the patient are indicative. Pathologic fractures, a frequent complication, may be subtle. There may also be blood or blood products within the lesion, as demonstrated in this case by the hypointense irregular structure.

Case 25

Knee

History

This 65-year-old woman observed a slowly growing mass in the area of the right knee. She had no pain, but some restriction of movement. On clinical examination a well-circumscribed mass that is not fixed to the surface could be palpated. There were no skin changes and no other obvious clinical signs.

Imaging

1. Plain Film Radiographs

Fig. 25.1
Both knees,
a. p. projection

Plain film radiographs reveal a large, ovoid, rather homogeneous soft tissue density in the lateral aspect of the right knee, with a craniocaudal extension of at least 10 cm. There is no evidence of associated bone erosion, and no calcifications are obvious within the mass (Fig. 25.1).

2. Magnetic Resonance Imaging

Fig. 25.2
Right knee

a T1-SE, sagittal plane
b T1-SE after contrast
administration, axial
plane

Magnetic resonance imaging reveals a well-circumscribed ovoid mass ventrally and adjacent to the patellar ligament, starting at the level of the apex of the patella and extending caudally to the level of the tibial tuberosity. The mass is considered extraarticular with convex bowing of the skin ventrally, but with no signs of infiltration. The tumor has an craniocaudal diameter of ca. 7 cm and a transverse diameter of 4.5 × 2.5 cm. The high and rather homogeneous signal intensity on T1- and T2-SE images is equivalent to that of fat (Fig. 25.2a). After contrast medium administration there is no enhancement (Figs. 25.2b, c). There is a subtle septation in the superior aspect of the lesion.

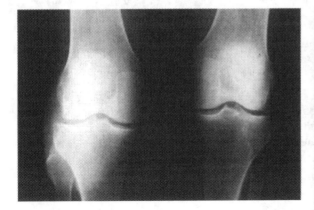

Fig. 25.1. Both knees, a.p. projection

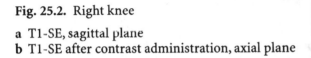

Fig. 25.2. Right knee

a T1-SE, sagittal plane
b T1-SE after contrast administration, axial plane

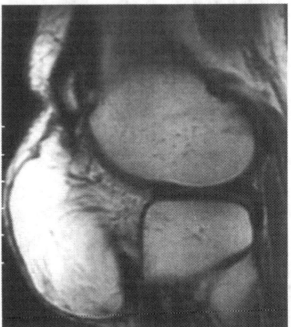

a

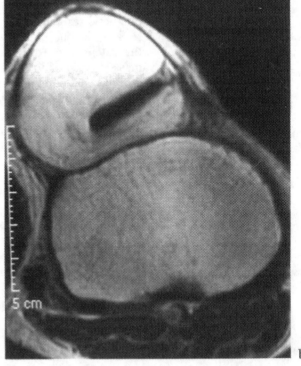

b

Why and What

1. Lipoma

There is a slowly growing, painless extraarticular mass anterior to the patellar ligament with signal characteristics isointense to fat on all image sequences. Despite the size of the lesion, these characteristics indicate a benign fat-containing tumor. The MRI characteristics of this lesion are pathognomonic. They fulfil the criteria for fat in all sequences, and there is evidence of a communication with Hoffa's fat pad, which further underlines the diagnosis.

2. Soft Tissue Tumor

Plain radiographs provide evidence of a large soft tissue tumor, but no further histologic conclusions can be drawn. Only a limited number of lesions can be excluded: a primary bony lesion, owing to the absence of any cortical or osseous change; a chondromatous tumor, owing to the absence of an cloud-like, partly calcified appearance of the matrix; and hemangioma, owing to the lack of calcifications and of clinical signs such as associated skin changes.

3. Atypical Lipoma, Liposarcoma

The only aspect that might cause some uncertainty is the size of the lesion, as well-differentiated liposarcomas may also be encapsulated. However, lipomas are the only soft tissue tumors which, even when greater than 5 cm in diameter, do not necessarily arouse suspicion of malignancy. As a general rule for fat-containing tumors, increasing inhomogenity, decreasing signal intensity on T1-weighted images and increasing signal intensity on T2-weighted images indicate malignancy.

On MRI, the signal characteristics depend on the amount of differentiation and correlate with the histologic subtypes with regard to the amount of mature fat present. Myxoid liposarcomas are encapsulated and usually septated; however, lower signal would be expected on T1-weighted images than in our case. Round-cell and pleomorphic subtypes would have a more heterogeneous appearance, and only types with a considerable amount of fatty tissue would show similar signal characteristics, but again with a less homogeneous appearance.

Atypical lipomas such as myxoid liposarcoma with an extracellular consisting of mature fat cells interspersed with multinucleated cells, collagen bundles, and adipocytes differ histologically from simple lipomas, and therefore also display a more inhomogeneous tumor matrix.

Final Diagnosis

Histologic Examination of the Surgical Specimen Confirmed the Diagnosis of Lipoma

Definition. Solitary lipomas consist entirely of mature fat. Lipomas are occasionally altered by the admixture of other mesenchymal elements lying inside the tumor. The most common of these structures is fibrous connective tissue which is often hyalinized and may or may not be associated with a capsule or the fibrous septum.

Incidence. The reported incidence of lipoma is probably much lower than the actual incidence. Nevertheless, lipoma represents the most common neoplasm of mesenchymal origin.

Age, sex distribution. Some report a higher incidence in men, others in women. Lipomas are rare during the first two decades of life. They appear mainly in the fifth and sixth decades.

Location. Two types of solitary lipomas are distinguished: superficial and deep-seated. The superficial type is most common in the back, shoulder, upper neck, and abdomen, followed by the proximal parts of the extremities. Deep-seated lipomas are rare in comparison. They are found in the mediastinum, the retroperitoneum, the chest wall, and the extremities.

Therapy. Marginal excision is the treatment of choice.

Prognosis. Lipomas are benign. They may recur locally after intralesional resection. Malignant transformation is extremely rare.

Case 26   Forefoot

History

A 41-year-old woman presented with a palpable mass on the plantar aspect of the right forefoot between the third and fourth toes. The patient reported that the lesion had been slowly growing over the last year, but she had suffered no pain. There were no skin changes and no other clinical signs.

Imaging

1. Plain Film Radiographs

Fig. 26.1
Right forefoot

a Lateral projection
b Lateral projection, enlarged
c Digits 3 and 4, a. p. projection

Plain film radiographs reveal cloud-like calcifications in the plantar plane of the forefoot, laterally from the proximal phalanx of the third toe (ca. 4 × 2 cm). There is an associated diffuse increase in soft tissue density around the area of the calcifications, extending proximally and distally. The calcifications in a small area seem adjacent to the cortical bone; however, there is no evidence of erosion or destruction, and the cortical bone can be delineated discerned in continuity.

2. Magnetic Resonance Imaging

Fig. 26.2
Right foot

a T1-SE, coronal plane
b T1-SE after contrast administration, axial plane

Magnetic resonance imaging reveals a soft tissue mass which extends between the third and fourth proximal phalangeal bones and in plantar disection into the plantar plate of the foot. The lesion has broad contact with the adjacent cortical bone, and shows a diameters of ca. 3 × 2 cm. It is hypointense on T1-weighted images and shows high signal characteristics on STIR images. The lesion is partly inhomogeneous with small areas of loss of signal intensity on all sequences, indicating calcifications. After administration of contrast medium no significant enhancement is obvious. In those areas in which the mass shows maximal contact with the adjacent cortical bone, thinning of the cortex might be suspected; however, no infiltration or destruction of bone is obvious, and the bone marrow shows regular signal characteristics. Concerning the extension towards the plantar plate, there is a moderate mass effect with some obliteration and displacement of the subcutaneous fat tissue.

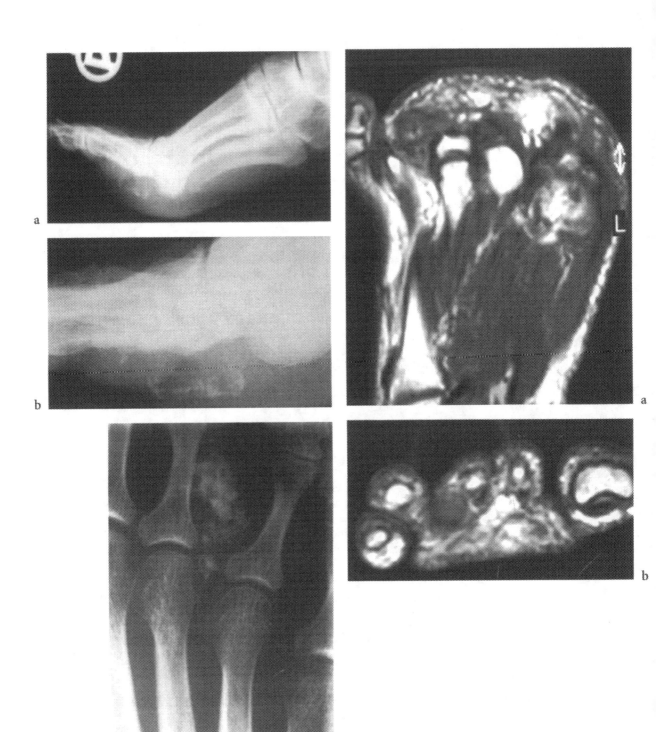

Differential Diagnosis Based on Radiographs

- Extraskeletal chondroma or osteochondroma
- Extraskeletal chondrosarcoma
- Myositis (Panniculitis) ossificans

Differential Diagnosis Based on Radiographs and Further Studies

- Extraskeletal chondroma
- Pseudomalignant osseous soft tissue tumor
- Myositis ossificans

Why and What

There is evidence of a calcified soft tissue mass in the plantar soft tissue compartment. The popcorn or cloud-like appearance of the calcification pattern is reminiscent of a chondromatous lesion. However, there is no evidence of a primarily osseous association. The lack of enhancement indicates only little biological activity and suggests a benign lesion.

1. Extraskeletal Chondroma or Osteochondroma

The cloud-like or popcorn-like calcification pattern is indicative of a chondromatous lesion. Although there is no evidence of a primarily osseous origin of the lesion, extraskeletal chondroma or osteochondroma is therefore our first diagnosis. The MRI patterns (T2 high signal) are consistent with a chondromatous lesion. As there is no significant enhancement after contrast medium administration we suspect a more benign lesion, as would be the case with extraskeletal chondroma.

2. Pseudomalignant Osseous Soft Tissue Tumor

This is a rare bone-forming soft tissue mass, with a predilection for the hands and feet. Tumors arise from the periosteum or fibrous septa, which might be assumed in the present case. The tumor grows slowly, up to a maximum size of 3 cm, and the MRI signal characteristics (low on T1-, inhomogeneous on T2-weighted sequences) would also be consistent. However, as the lesion occurs in young adults and adolescents, the age of our patient is not in addition, the potential periosteal reaction is absent, as is the characteristic appearance of a zone phenomenon with peripheral mature bone.

3. Myositis Ossificans

Myositis ossificans is a benign, heterotopic soft tissue ossification and may result from several different causes. Frequently it occurs following trauma or in the course of an underlying neurologic disease, neither of which was reported by this patient. The ectopic bone usually lies longitudinally along the axis of muscle, what is not evident in our case. The MRI patterns depend on the age and maturation of the lesion. Although the signal characteristics are not specific, in our case they could possibly be consistent with myositis ossificans.

Final Diagnosis

Extraskeletal Chondroma

Definition. Neoformation of well-differentiated hyaline cartilage, which is often associated with tendons, tendon sheaths, or joint capsule, but is clearly outside the joint. Furthermore it is unlike periosteal chondroma in that it is located outside the periosteum.

Age, sex distribution. The tumor affects adults between 30 and 60 years of age. There is no gender predilection.

Location. Eighty percent of extraskeletal chondromas are found in the fingers; less frequent sites are the hands, toes, feet, and trunk.

Therapy. Marginal excision.

Prognosis. In the case of intralesional resection local recurrence may occur.

Case 27   Knee, Thigh

History

This 18-year-old woman reported a 4-month history of increasing pain and soft tissue swelling in the right thigh. Clinically the pain increased with physical pressure. No other symptoms were evident.

Imaging

1. Plain Film Radiographs

Fig. 27.1
Right knee and distal femur, a. p. projection

A soft tissue swelling can be observed in the right thigh. Small calcifications can be suspected within the soft tissue. Cortical thickening in this area is clearly seen, but there is no further evidence of associated bony lesion. The knee joint is normal (Fig. 27.1).

2. Magnetic Resonance Imaging

Fig. 27.2
Right knee and distal femur

a T1-SE, coronal plane
b T1-SE after contrast administration, coronal plane
c T1-SE after contrast administration, axial plane

Magnetic resonance imaging reveals a mass in a periosseous location around the distal third of the femur. The lesion has broad contact with the cortical bone in the lateral aspect of the femur and surrounds the femur for about 180° (Fig. 27.2a). The maximum width of the lesion is 1.5 cm, and the maximal craniocaudal diameter is 4.5 cm. On T1-SE images the lesion shows inhomogeneous, mainly low signal intensities and is demarcated from the surrounding muscles by a fat plane (Fig. 27.2b). On T2-SE images the lesion demonstrates worm-like hyperintensities. The lesion shows a mass effect on the surrounding structures; however, there is no evidence of invasion. There are also no signs of destruction of the adjacent cortical bone. After administration of a gadolinium-containing agent there is moderate inhomogeneous enhancement of signal intensities, with a partly cloudy and partly streaky appearance. A tubular area of contrast enhancement might be suspected (Figs. 27.2a, c).

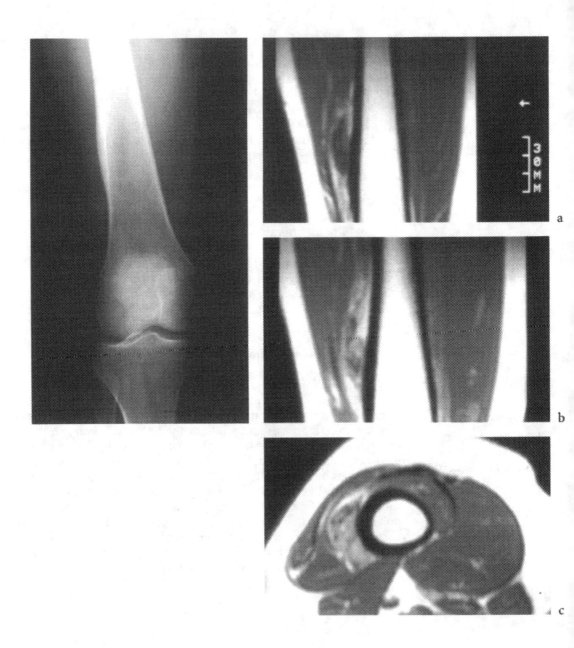
a

b

c

Why and What

1. Hemangioma

Hemanioma is always suspected in a soft tissue lesion with evidence of calcifications. The signal characteristics on MRI reinforce the suspicion by demonstrating a worm-like appearance of the lesion with evidence of both fast (flow void: no signal) and slow (hyperintense tubular) blood flow representing the vascular structure of a hemangioma. After administration of contrast medium enhancement of some parts of the lesion may be observed, indicating venous flow. These observations fulfil the criteria for a vascularized, non-infiltrative, slowly growing benign tumor such as hemangioma.

2. Myositis Ossificans

Myositis ossificans usually occurs in young adults, and chronic trauma or other underlying disease such as hemophilia or neurologic conditions may be found in the history, which is not the case here. Although the ectopic bone usually lies longitudinally to the axis of the muscle, the adjacent periosteum may react. From plain film radiographs the diagnosis of myositis ossificans therefore cannot be excluded. MRI, however, depending on the age and maturation of the lesion, show patterns of edema and hemorrhage, whereas the calcification remains hypointense on T1- and T2-weighted images. However, the worm-like pattern in this case, together with signal characteristics indicating blood flow, is not compatible with the diagnosis of myositis ossificans.

3. Soft Tissue Tumor

Other soft tissue tumors might have MRI characteristics resembling those here; however, only rarely would they show calcifications. Soft tissue tumors with inhomogeneous T2 hyperintensities are: malignant fibrous histiocytoma, synovial sarcoma, alveolar sarcoma, rhabdomyosarcoma, and epitheloid sarcoma. None of these tumors, however, typically shows calcifications, which might be expected only in chronic disease.

4. Inflammatory Process

The MRI findings might also be consistent with a periosseous chronic soft tissue inflammation. However, there are no signs of bone marrow edema, which would be expected. Also the calcifications would only be expected late in a prolonged course of disease.

Final Diagnosis

Intramuscular Hemangioma with Metaplastic Ossifications

Definition. Hemangioma is essentially defined as a benign but nonreactive process in which there is an increase in the number of normal or abnormal vessels. This benign lesion is difficult to distinguish from neoplasm, hamartoma, or malformation. It occurs as localized hemangioma or as diffuse hemangioma, termed angiomatosis. The localized form is classified into capillary hemangioma, cavernous hemangioma, venous hemangioma, arteriovenous hemangioma, epitheloid hemangioma, and miscellaneous hemangiomas of the deep soft tissue (synovial, intramuscular, neural), primarily based on pathologic changes. In this case the lesion is a deep-seated intramuscular hemangioma.

Incidence. The intramuscular form is the most common type of deep-seated hemangioma but represents only 8% of all benign vascular tumors.

Age, sex distribution. The majority of intramuscular hemangiomas occur in young adults, 80–90% before the age of 30 years. If arising early, the lesion may be of congenital origin. The male to female ratio is 1:1.

Location. Although any muscle can be affected, the majority of such hemangiomas are located in the lower extremity, particularly in the muscles of the thigh.

Therapy. Complete excision or repeated embolization, sometimes prior to surgical excision.

Remarks

Calcifications in a soft tissue mass, together with the clinical signs and the age of the patient, are almost specific for hemangioma. The ossifications are due to phleboliths in small vessels within the hemangioma. MRI demonstrates worm-like hyperintensity on T2-SE images with hypointense phleboliths on T1- and T2-SE images and enhancement after contrast medium administration, indicating the vascularized nature of the tumor. Note that enhancement of the lesion may be delayed, or not visible, if the postcontrast images are obtained immediately after contrast administration. Therefore, delayed postcontrast images might be helpful in questionable cases.

Most hemangioma are of the capillary-cavernous type. This is important for the differential diagnosis where fast-flow and slow-flow lesions can be differentiated by evaluation of the first-pass dynamic contrast enhancement.

Case 28   Pelvis

History

This 35-year-old man had already undergone surgery for a cartilaginous exostosis in early childhood. He experienced no symptoms until 4 months before presentation, when he observed a growing mass in the left pelvis. On palpation the mass was firm and could not be moved. There was no soft tissue swelling, and the skin in the area was normal. The patient reported only moderate pain.

Imaging

1. Plain Film Radiographs

Fig. 28.1

a Pelvis, a. p. projection
b Distal femur,
   a. p. projection
c Left knee joint and
   proximal tibia, lateral
   projection

Plain film radiographs of the pelvis (ap view) reveal a huge cloudy mass in the area of the left pelvis with a diameter of 11 × 12 cm. The regular bone is totally destroyed and replaced by bizarre calcifications which demonstrate a cloud-like appearance. The border of the mass is ill defined; however, it only partly exceeds the previous contours of the iliac bone (Fig. 28.1 a).

Several other lesions are obvious: One arises from the medial dorsal aspect of the iliac crest and has a mushroom-like appearance with a diameter of 6 × 5 cm. It is a bony mass with an irregular, partly lucent pattern and a streaky, irregularly calcified matrix. The border of the lesion can be discerned. A similar lesion arises from the minor tubercle of the left femur (5 × 3 cm), and a smaller lesion can be observed in the area of the left femur which is predominantly radiolucent and shows a thin cortical border (Fig. 28.1 b).

Plain film radiographs of the knee further demonstrate a huge epimetaphyseal mass in the left proximal tibia, which displays a prominent, cloud-like calcification centrally and polypoid well-defined margins. This mass also arises from the underlying bone (Fig. 28.1 c).

2. Magnetic Resonance Imaging

Fig. 28.2
Pelvis

a T1-SE, axial plane
b T1-SE after contrast
   administration, axial
   plane
c T2-SE, axial plane

MRI of the pelvis demonstrates the mass in the left iliac bone as a huge hypointense area with a smaller part in the iliac bone and a huge part that extends dorsally and laterally and reaches the subcutaneous fat tissue. The muscles in this area can no longer be detected in their regular anatomic position. The lesion is hypointense on T1-weighted images (Fig. 28.2 a) and demonstrates only minimal enhancement after administration of contrast medium (Fig. 28.2 b). On T2-weighted images, however, the lesion has confluent hyperintense signal characteristics which in part even resemble the signal intensity of fluid (Fig. 28.2 c). The lesion is well circumscribed, and there is no evidence of involvement of the adjacent soft tissue. There is also no sign of a bone marrow reaction or edema in the remaining normal-appearing marrow of the iliac bone.

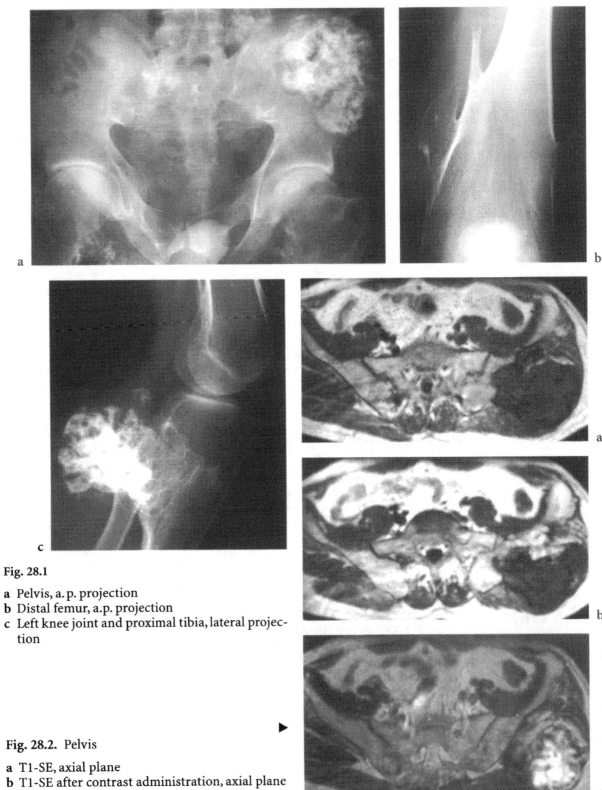

Fig. 28.1

a Pelvis, a. p. projection
b Distal femur, a.p. projection
c Left knee joint and proximal tibia, lateral projection

Fig. 28.2. Pelvis

a T1-SE, axial plane
b T1-SE after contrast administration, axial plane
c T2-SE, axial plane

Differential Diagnosis Based on Radiographs

- Multiple cartilaginous exostoses with malignant transformation to chondrosarcoma
- Basically same diagnosis with malignant transformation to osteosarcoma
- Basically same diagnosis with malignant transformation to fibrosarcoma

Differential Diagnosis Based on Radiographs and Further Studies

- Chondrosarcoma
- Fibrosarcoma
- Osteosarcoma

Why and What

1. Malignant Transformation of Cartilaginous Exostoses to Chondrosarcoma

There are multiple exostotic lesions in this patient, and due to the evident history of surgery for a cartilaginous exostoses in the patients childhood, the diagnosis of the lesions in both femurs and the knee must be that of multiple cartilaginous exostoses, which is supported by a classic mushroom-like exostotic appearance. However, the lesion in the left iliac bone gives cause for concern. It shows an amorphous cloud-like and calcified appearance with ill-defined borders and it is huge. Therefore we have to consider the possibility of an underlying malignancy in this lesion. The amorphous huge calcifications, the irregularity of the borders, and the apparent destruction of the underlying bone strongly suggest malignant transformation of an underlying cartilaginous exostosis in a case of hereditary multiple exostoses. We note particularly the destruction at the base of the lesion, which is a definite sign of malignancy. The most frequent type of malignant transformation is that into chondrosarcoma. The cartilaginous parts demonstrate high signal intensity on T2-weighted images, which is also evident in our case. Moreover, the cloud-like or popcorn like appearance on plain film radiographs gives strong evidence of an chondromatous matrix.

2. Fibrosarcoma, Osteosarcoma

Another possibility is that of malignant transformation into a fibrosarcoma or osteosarcoma. The lesion shows very little enhancement after contrast medium administration, which might indicate a very fibrous or calcified tissue; however, the confluent high signal intensities on T2-weighted images are more indicative of an chondromatous than a fibrous matrix. Osteosarcoma potentially could demonstrate similar signal characteristics; however, we might expect more destruction of the underlying bone and/or more adjacent soft tissue or bone marrow reaction.

Final Diagnosis

Chondrosarcoma Arising from Multiple Hereditary Cartilaginous Exostoses

Multiple cartilaginous exostoses are characterized by three main aspects:

1. Heredity
2. Association with skeletal shortening and deformity
3. Frequent transformation into peripheral chondrosarcoma

Incidence. The ratio of multiple to solitary exostoses is about 1:10.

Age, sex distribution. Multiple exostoses generally are manifested before the age of 10 years.
There is a predilection for males (ratio 2:1).

Location. Multiple exostoses are generally diffuse and relatively symmetrical. They may occur in all bones, arising from cartilage. Generally exostoses are more frequent, larger and develop in all metaphysis of the upper and lower limb.

Therapy. Not all of the exostoses can be removed; however, generally those that cause pressure or deformity or are located in the central parts of the body are surgically removed.

Remarks

Solitary osteocartilaginous exostosis (i.e., osteochondroma) is a bony projection with a cartilaginous cap. The cortex is continuous with the cortex of the parent bone, as is the periosteum. It usually forms at the metaphysis of a tubular bone. Hereditary multiple exostosis is characterized by multiple osteochondromas. There are four distinct forms of osteochondromas: pedunculated, sessile, calcific, and giant:
The pedunculated form is an osteocartilaginous cap on a long, narrow base. The sessile form is broad-based without an elongated projection, forming a local widening of the shaft of the bone. The radiologic hallmark of both types is the continuity of the cortex of the osteochondroma with the cortex of the normal bone. The cap shows irregularity, and the cartilage may calcify extensively with an amorphous spotty appearance. MRI can demonstrate anatomic relations and assess the thickness of the cartilaginous cap. MR imaging allows visualization of the cap, which shows high signal intensity on T2-weighted images, and measurement of its thickness. A band of low signal intensity represents the perichondrium. Malignant transformation may be suspected if growth takes place in a previously stable lesion. Extensive calcification may be present in a benign lesion, but a large associated soft tissue mass that contains streaky calcification should be suspected of being malignant. A soft tissue mass with a thickness greater than 2 cm on CT or MRI should arouse suspicion of a malignancy. Invasion and destruction of the base of the osteochondroma are definite signs of chondrosarcomatous change.

Case 29   Proximal Femur

History

This 54-year-old man presented with a soft tissue mass in the right upper thigh. The lesion had been evident for 8 months and had increased in size. There is only mild pain, and no skin alterations are evident. Palpation reveals a firm indolent mass.

Imaging

1. Plain Film Radiographs

Fig. 29.1
Right proximal femur,
a. p. projection

Plain film radiographs reveal a soft tissue density in the anterior aspect of the right upper thigh. There is no evidence of associated bone destruction, and no calcifications are evident within the soft tissue mass (Fig. 29.1).

2. Magnetic Resonance Imaging

Fig. 29.2
Right thigh

a T1-SE, parasagittal
plane
b T1-SE after contrast
administration,
parasagittal plane
c T1-SE after contrast
administration, axial
plane

Magnetic resonance imaging reveals a mass in the area of the sartorius muscle. The mass has an diameter of 13 × 6 × 4 cm (craniocaudal × axial × transverse) (Figs. 29.2a, b). The lesion is rather well defined with smooth borders. There is a fat plane separating the mass from the adjacent muscles, with only some irregular appearance of the otherwise smooth border in the most caudal aspect of the lesion. The lesion shows a mass effect with moderate displacement of the dorsally adjacent muscle groups; however, there is no evidence of infiltration. The femoral nerve, running alongside the vascular bundle, comes close to the mass, but seems separated from it by the fat plane (Fig. 29.2c). After administration of contrast medium there is strong enhancement of the tumor, particularly in the peripheral parts, whereas nonenhancing irregular areas remain in the central parts of the tumor (Fig. 29.2c). No other lesions are evident; particularly, the femur is clearly distant from the lesion, shows regular signal characteristics and is not affected.

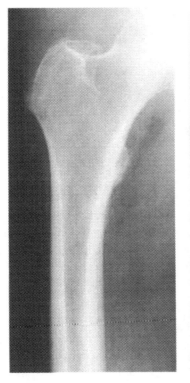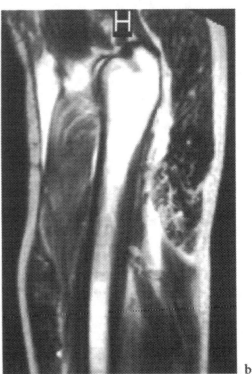

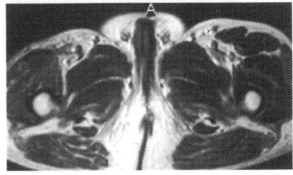

b

c

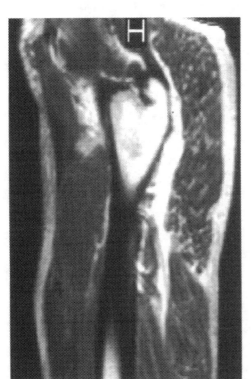

Differential Diagnosis Based on Radiographs

- Soft tissue tumor
- Posttraumatic soft tissue swelling
- Chronic inflammatory process

Differential Diagnosis Based on Radiographs and Further Studies

- Soft tissue tumor
- Malignant fibrous histiocytoma
- Rhabdomyosarcoma
- Soft tissue metastases

Why and What

1. Soft Tissue Tumor

There is a large tumor arising from the soft tissue of the anterior compartment of the upper thigh. Although the tumor seems well defined and expansive rather than infiltrative, its size and enhancement patterns are strongly suggestive of a malignant lesion. There is no cortical destruction or involvement of the bones, indicating a primary or secondary soft tissue tumor. From plain film radiographs alone only a vague differential diagnosis can be made. A soft tissue tumor is most probable, as there are no clinical signs indicating any inflammatory process, and there is also no evidence of trauma. In both inflammation and trauma a soft tissue swelling might be observed. The absence of involvement of the adjacent bone leads us to the suspicion of a primary soft tissue tumor. There are no obvious calcifications, which, together with the age of the patient, only let us exclude the diagnosis of hemangioma.

Angiography demonstrates atypical feeding vessels, together with an arched appearance. This is indicative of a probably malignant soft tissue tumor. The nature of the tumor cannot be narrowed down further.

2. Malignant Fibrous Histiocytoma

Malignant fibrous histiocytoma is one of the most frequent malignant soft tissue tumor. The tumor is well vascularized and shows central necrotic parts, which underlines its malignant character.

3. Rhabdomyosarcoma

The tumor arises from muscle tissue, and indeed rhabdomyosarcoma might show the same imaging pattern and would radiologically be indistinguishable from any other fast-growing malignant soft tissue tumor.

4. Metastases

A soft tissue metastasis with central necrotic areas could potentially demonstrate an identical imaging pattern.

Final Diagnosis

Malignant Fibrous Histiocytoma

Definition. MFH is constituted by cells originating from histiocytic and fibro-blastic differentiation. Nowadays five entities of this tumor are distinguished:

1. Storiform pleomorphic
2. Myxoid
3. Giant-cell
4. Inflammatory
5. Angiomatoid

The different subtypes have different prognoses.

Incidence. MFH is one of the most frequently occuring malignant soft tissue tumors.

Age, sex distribution. The tumor appears in late adult life, except the angioma-toid form, which is manifested in the first and second decades of life.
There is an evident predilection for males.

Location. There is a preference for the lower limb and the retroperitoneum. Some 90% of all cases show a deep-seated tumor, while 10% are superficial. The angiomatoid MFH affects more the dermis and the subcutaneous tissue of the limbs.

Therapy. Wide or radical resection followed by irradiation and chemotherapy.

Prognosis. The prognosis depends mainly on clinical factors such as site, size, and location of the tumor. The more distal and the more superficial the tumor, the better the prognosis. Metastases are of MFH localized in the lungs (80%), lymph nodes (10%), liver, and bone.

Remarks

Basically MFH cannot be distinguished on radiological patterns from any other malignant soft tissue tumor; however, it is the most common tumor in adult life. The importance of neighboring structures such as the neurovascu-lar bundle and the femoral nerve and its relation to the the tumor, must be borne in mind when deciding on the surgical approach. Although the femoral nerve is of reduced visibility, its presence and relation to the tumor can be evaluated from its anatomic course.

Case 30   Midfoot

History

This 66-year-old man presented with a mass in the dorsal aspect of the first metatarsophalangeal joint. He had observed slow growth of the lesion for 8 months. The patient had only little pain; on palpation the mass is firm and not moveable. There are no skin changes and no evidence of other lesions.

Imaging

1. Plain Film Radiographs

Fig. 30.1
Right forefoot,
a. p. projection

Plain film radiographs reveal a soft tissue mass adjacent to the first metatarsophalangeal joint. There is no evidence of bony erosion, and there are no calcifications (Fig. 30.1).

2. Magnetic Resonance Imaging

Fig. 30.2
First metatarsopha-
langeal joint

a T1-SE, sagittal plane
b T1-SE after contrast
  administration, sagittal
  plane
c STIR, sagittal plane

T1-weighted images reveal a rather well circumscribed but inhomogeneous mass with an extent of ca. $5 \times 2 \times 2$ cm (Fig. 30.2a) at the first metatarsophalangeal joint. The lesion is basically hypointense but demonstrates streaky areas of hyperintense signal intensities, which are most prominent just next to the surface where the lesion shows a pseudocapsulated configuration. The axis of the lesion is parallel to the axis of the long bones and tendons. Those parts of the extensor hallucis longus tendon within the area of the lesion cannot be delineated, but the tendon show a regular configuration proximally and distally. On three sections the lesion has little, yet evident contact with the joint space, and an invasion can be suspected. Otherwise, on its undersurface, the lesion has broad contact with the adjacent bone. There might be some thinning of the corticalis, but there is no evidence of erosion or destruction. After contrast medium administration there is inhomogeneous moderate enhancement with a smaller unenhancing area centrally (Fig. 30.2b). Fat-suppressed STIR images reveal inhomogeneous hyperintense signal characteristics (Fig. 30.2c). There is a small subchondral hyperintense zone in the head of the metacarpal bone, but otherwise the bone marrow is regular. There is little joint fluid.

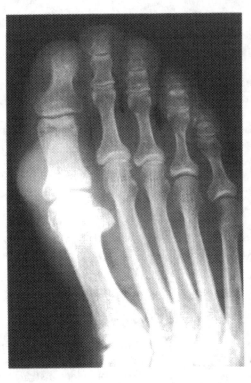

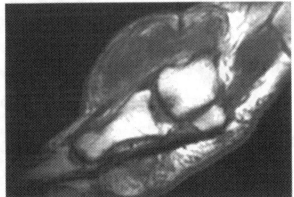

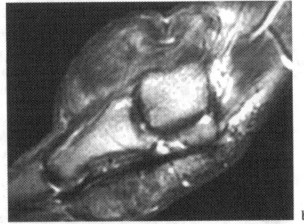

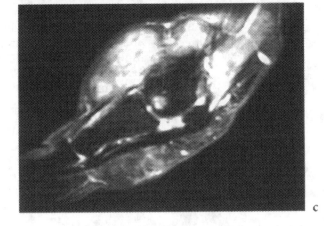

Differential Diagnosis Based on Radiographs

– Soft tissue tumor
– Inflammatory (rheumatoid) process

Differential Diagnosis Based on Radiographs and Further Studies

– Giant-cell tumor of the tendon sheath, pigmented villonodular synovitis
– Benign fibrous soft tissue tumor or low-grade malignant fibrous tumor
– Organized older abscess formation

Why and What

1. Giant Cell Tumor of the Tendon Sheath

There is an inhomogeneous soft tissue mass adjacent to the dorsal aspect of the first metatarsophalangeal joint. There is broad contact with the extensor hallucis tendon, which cannot be clearly delineated from the mass. There is no evidence of an associated osseous affection and no definite cortical destruction; however, there may be extension into the joint. Signal characteristics indicate a more fibrous yet inhomogeneous lesion, and the enhancement patterns indicates low to moderate biological activity. Due to its location we might suspect a lesion arising from those structures adjacent to the joint, namely the tendon and the synovial and perisynovial tissue. The matrix of the tumor does not show a typical chondromatous character, and a primary osseous lesion appears less probable.

Location and signal characteristics are consistent with the diagnosis of a giant-cell tumor of the tendon sheath. The lesion seems to be extraarticular, but shows close contact with the tendon. The signal characteristics would also be consistent with a more fibrous kind of tumor. The low signal intensity on T2-weighted images could be due to diffuse hemosiderin deposition and fibrous tissue.

2. Soft Tissue Tumor

Actually a variety of soft tissue tumors might show similar signal characteristics and enhancement patterns. However, we can fairly confidently exclude a chondromatous tumor, e.g., extraarticular chondromatosis, and also lipoma and hemangioma owing to the signal characteristics. The low enhancement and the low signal intensity on T2-weighted images indicate a more benign character of the lesion.

3. Rheumatoid Process, Older Inflammatory Process, Gout

The signal characteristics might also be considered to resemble an older encapsulated formation of inflammatory origin, as may appear in a gout tophus. However, there is no evidence of any involvement of the adjacent bone, there is no enhancement of the pseudocapsule, and the patient's history and clinical course tend to speak against to this diagnosis.

Final Diagnosis

Giant-Cell Tumor of the Tendon Sheath

See case 21

Definition. Hyperplastic production of synovial tissue of joints, tendon sheaths, bursae or fibrous tissue adjacent to the tendons. PVNS may be present in two manifestations:

- Diffuse villonodular form
- Localized nodular form

Synonyms. Xanthoma, xanthogranuloma, benign synovialoma, giant-cell tumor of the tendon sheath, fibrous histiocytoma of the synovium.

Incidence. The paratendineous nodular synovitis is particularly frequent in the hand. Joint affections are relatively rare.

Age, sex distribution. The highest incidence is between 20 and 40 years of age, but the range is 10–75 years. There is no gender predilection.

Location. PVNS is frequently observed in the fingers, where it occurs in the sheath of the flexor tendons. It is not very common in the foot in relation to the flexor and extensor tendons. Of the joints, more than 75% of all cases occur in the knee, followed by the hip, wrist, ankle, and shoulder.

Therapy. In the localized nodular form marginal excision is easy and, if it is completely performed, there is no recurrence. In the diffuse villonodular form, complete surgical excision may be difficult or impossible. There is a high risk of local recurrence.

Remarks

Pigmented villonodular synovitis, idiopathic synovial chondromatosis and infection are among the monoarticular processes that may be found in the foot and ankle. Because of the proximity to the adjacent tendon sheaths, a variety of lesions involving such sheaths can extend into a joint. These processes include tenosynovial chondromatosis, PVNS, and septic tenosynovitis.
Giant-cell tumors of soft tissue may arise from tendon sheaths as well as from joint capsules and ligamentous tissue. A mass with or without erosions of the subjacent bone and without calcification is evident. The relationship of giant-cell tumors of the tendon sheet to diffuse or localized pigmented villonodular synovitis is not clear, although the tumors may contain hemosiderin deposits. Owing to the presence of hemosiderin deposition or dense acellular fibrous tissue, the lesion may be of low signal intensity on both T1- and T2-weighted SE images.

Cave: Metatarsophalangeal Joint

Case 31　Clavicle

History

This 76-year-man recognized a growing tumor in the right sternoclavicular region 7 months before presentation. The palpable painless lesion now measured 5–6 cm. No other lesions could be found.

Imaging

1. Plain Film Radiographs

Fig. 31.1
Right clavicle

At the sternal end of the right clavicle caudally there is a cortical irregularity, but no calcifications. The neighboring spongiosa is within normal limits (Fig. 31.1).

2. Ultrasound

Fig. 31.2
Right clavicle, sonographic appearance of the tumor

The palpable tumor mass is well delineated, solid and homogeneous with low echogenicity. It measures about 3–4 cm (Fig. 31.2).

3. Magnetic Resonance Imaging

Fig. 31.3
Upper thoracic aperture

a T1-SE, axial plane
b T1-SE after contrast administration, axial plane

On T1-SE images the lesion is homogeneous with low signal intensity (Fig. 31.3a). It is well delineated and enhances homogeneously after i. v. contrast injection (Fig. 31.3b) The sternal end of the right clavicle touches directly the tumor.

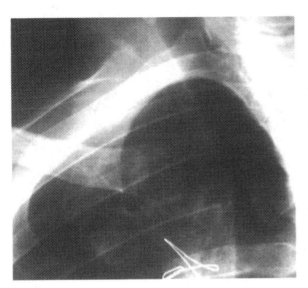

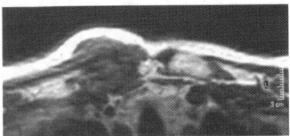

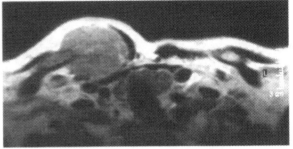

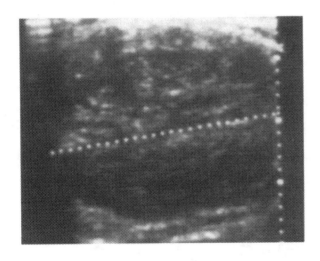

Why and What

1. Plasmocytoma

Plasmocytomas arise from the bone marrow and lead primarily to an osteolytic lesion. In our case a soft tissue tumor is infiltrating the adjacent bone!

2. Lymphoma

Primary lymphomas of the soft tissue are commonly non-Hodgkin lymphoma. These are solid soft tissue masses which may show central necrosis, if they are large enough. Otherwise the lesions are homogeneous and enhance after i.v. injection of contrast medium. Non-Hodgkin lymphoma may grow diffusely and infiltrate surrounding tissues, such as the bone in our case.

3. Metastasis

In this age group a metastasis should be always a differential diagnosis. In this case no primary tumor is known, and it is also uncommon to find soft-tissue metastases as the primary manifestation of a carcinoma. Metastasis cannot be ruled out, however.

Final Diagnosis

B-Cell Non-Hodgkin Lymphoma (Low Malignancy)

Definition. Hodgkin lymphoma and non-Hodgkin Lymphoma (NHL), are malignant tumors which generally speaking can arise from any cells of the lymphoreticular tissue. Most of them, however, arise from immunocompetent cells. Lymphomas are differentiated by B- or T-cell origin; low, intermediate, and high malignancy; and by their origin from precursor or peripheral cells. A definite assignment of tumor cells for Hodgkin disease into the lymphocytic maturation rank until now could not be found.

Clinical manifestation. Low-malignant NHL has the following characteristics: slow growth (also without therapy), usually advanced stage at time of diagnosis, good response to low aggressive chemotherapy.
The most frequent clinical manifestations are painless swelling of lymph nodes in the axilla and inguinal sites. Weight reduction, sweat attacks and general symptoms may appear.

Therapy. In localized manifestations local radiation therapy shows good results. In advanced stages, if the patient is in good clinical condition a "wait and see policy" may be followed, or the initiation of systemic chemotherapy is indicated. In younger patients stem-cell transplantations are performed.

Case 32   Fibula, Lower Leg

History

This 55-year-old oligophrenic woman had recognized a tumor in her left axilla 3 months previously. The tumor was removed and histologically identified as a metastasis of an unknown primary. For about 4–6 weeks she had experienced pain and swelling in her right calf.

Clinical examination showed a large tumor within the calf and diffuse swelling of the ankle. There were some signs of inflammation.

Imaging

1. Plain Film Radiographs

Fig. 32.1
Right lower leg,
a.p. projection

In the middle third of the fibula there is a 8-cm-long area of permeative and lytic bony destruction where the bone structures have largely disappeared. There may be minute periosteal new bone formations at the lower end with some reactive medullary sclerosis outside the destructive lesion.

The soft tissue of the whole lower leg seems swollen and dense. There are some vascular calcifications (Fig. 32.1).

2. Magnetic Resonance Imaging

Fig. 32.2
Right lower leg

a T1-SE, axial plane
b T1-SE after contrast administration with fat suppression (SPIR), axial plane
c T1-SE after contrast administration with fat suppression (SPIR), coronal plane

A huge tumor mass (about $10 \times 8 \times 8$ cm) with almost complete destruction of the fibula in the involved part is revealed. The tumor is hypointense on T1-SE images (Fig. 32.2a) and demonstrates extensive, inhomogeneous enhancement after administration of contrast medium, with several areas remaining unenhanced (Figs. 32.2b, c). The surface of the tumor is in part regular, but irregular in the dorsomedial aspect. The main vessels are displaced, compressed, and reveal hyperintensity, probably because of slow flow or thrombosis. On the postcontrast images numerous ectatic venous vessels are seen (Figs. 32.2a, b). The bony structures of the tibia are well preserved, the cortex is intact, and the fatty marrow displays no abnormalities.

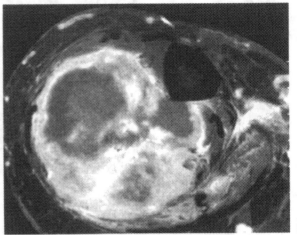

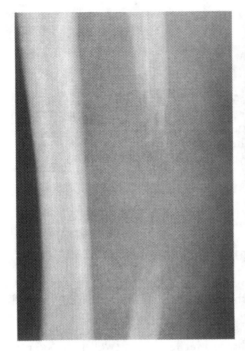

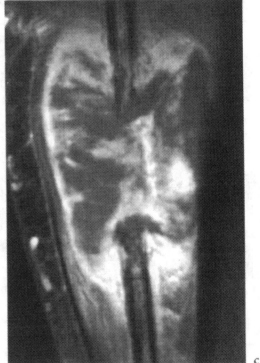

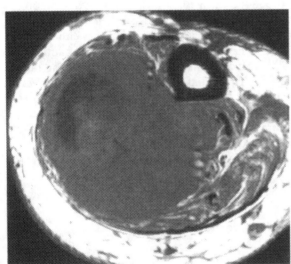

Differential Diagnosis Based on Radiographs

– Metastasis
– Lymphoma
– Plasmocytoma

Differential Diagnosis Based on Radiographs and Further Studies

– Metastasis
– Lymphoma/plasmo-
  cytoma
– Malignant fibrous
  histiocytoma

Why and What

1. Metastasis

Metastatic lesions in the fibula are rare. Osteolytic lesions represent about 75% of all metastases. The primary tumors are usually in the breast, lung, kidney, GI tract or thyroid. In a patient over the age of 50 years the first differential diagnosis in a destructive bone lesion must always be metastasis.

2. Lymphoma/Plasmocytoma

Lymphoma has a peak incidence between 35 and 60 years. The lesion may be geographic, moth-eaten, or permeative. There is almost never periosteal new bone formation. Sometimes non-Hodgkin lymphoma, more often Hodgkin lymphomas, has an ivory appearance (particularly in the vertebrae or flat bones). Hodgkin lymphomas are more typically found in bones where red marrow is present, while non-Hodgkin lymphomas are rarely found within bones, so a lymphoma is very unlikely within the fibula.
Lymphomas are usually homogeneous and show strong enhancement after i. v. contrast medium injection.
In our case – if the previous axillary lymph node metastasis had not been known – a lymphoma would be a possible albeit unlikely consideration.

3. Malignant Fibrous Histiocytoma

Malignant fibrous histiocytoma of the fibula is rare. The bony abnormalities as visualized in our case – osteolysis with permeative pattern – are found in MFH. Also the lack of reactive periosteal bone formation is characteristical. MFH occurs between the ages of 20 and 60 years. MFH may show a lot of necrotic tissue.

Final Diagnosis

Metastasis of a Solid, Polymorphous-Cellular Carcinoma

Definition. Metastases are secundary manifestations of a primary tumor.

Frequency. Metastases are the most frequent malignant tumors of the skeleton. If clinical and radiologic material is evaluated, about 15% of all carcinomas have skeletal manifestations. In autopsy material this can increase to 30%. Most metastases in bones are from primary tumors of five organs: breast, prostata, lung, kidney, thyroid.

Age, sex distribution. Generally speaking, bony lesions in patients over the age of 40 must be suspected to be metastases.

Location. There is an evident predilection for the skeleton of the trunk and the limb girdles. The tumors are principally localized in the vertebral column, the pelvis, and the upper ends of humerus and femur. They rarely occur distal to the elbow and knee.

Therapy. Surgical treatment is almost always palliative. Nerve root decompression, spinal cord decompression, surgical stabilization, osteosynthesis with screw fixation and acrylic cement, or, in rare cases, a tumor endoprosthesis is chosen depending on the clinical symptoms. Alternatives are selective arterial embolization, radiotherapy, chemotherapy, and hormone therapy. Therapy planning for bone metastases is truly interdisciplinary, involving oncologists, orthopedic surgeons, other specialist surgeons, radiotherapists, and others.

Prognosis. In many cases the disease is fatal; when bone metastases occur, survival generally drops to 1–2 years. Nevertheless, with the help of chemotherapy the overall survival is steadily increasing.

Case 33   Pelvis

History

This 61-year-old woman had suffered pain in the left hip while walking for 4 months. There was no trauma. Clinical examination revealed no signs of inflammation or joint effusion.

Imaging

1. Plain Film Radiographs

Fig. 33.1
Pelvis, a. p. projection

Radiographs of the pelvis demonstrate a well-demarcated lytic lesion in the area of the left anterior superior iliac spine. The lesion has a partially sclerotic margin medially, caudally, and cranially. Only the lateral rim is irregular, fuzzy, and partly destroyed (Fig. 33.1). Laterally and caudally adjacent to the lytic lesion, there is a soft tissue mass with a diameter of 3 – 5 cm and tiny irregular calcifications. No other lesions are discerned; in particular, the left hip and sacroiliac joint are within normal limits.

The multiple oval-shaped calcifications within the minor pelvis are probably phleboliths.

2. Magnetic Resonance Imaging

Fig. 33.2
Left iliac bone

a T2-weighted proton density image, coronal plane
b T1-SE after contrast administration, axial plane

T1-weighted SE images demonstrates a lobulated hypointense mass with an intraosseous part and a pedunculated extraosseous part. On T2-weighted images the lesion has intermediate signal intensities with some punctate inhomogeneities (Fig. 33.2a). The craniocaudal dimension of the mass is 6 cm and it extends into the supraacetabular region. There is no evidence of infiltration of the hip joint. In the axial plane the tumor has a large extraosseous pedunculated component at its lateral aspect and shows broad communication with the medullary cavity of the iliac bone. The axial diameters are about 3×3.5 cm. Axial T1-weighted images after contrast medium administration demonstrate rather homogeneous enhancement of the lesion (Fig. 33.2b). The extraosseous component is generally well delineated, with only some irregularity to the gluteus muscle, but does not show a hypointense sclerotic rim. The intraosseous component indicates scalloping with thinning and bowing of the adjacent cortex; however, destruction is only observed laterally.

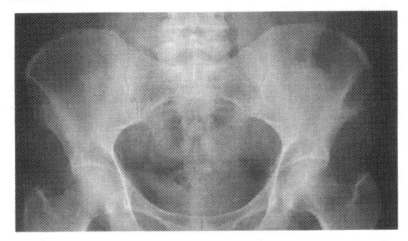

Fig. 33.1. Pelvis, a. p. projection
◀

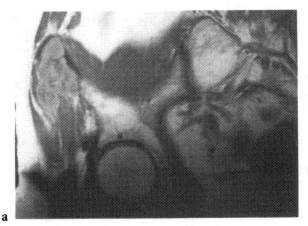

a

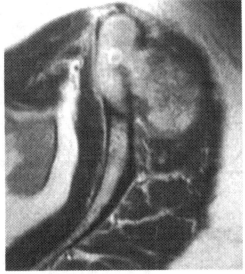

b

Fig. 33.2. Left iliac bone

a T2-weighted proton density image, coronal plane
b T1-SE after contrast administration, axial plane

Differential Diagnosis Based on Radiographs

- Chondrosarcoma
- Osteosarcoma
- Metastases

Differential Diagnosis Based on Radiographs and Further Studies

- Osteochondroma with malignant transformation
- Periosteal osteosarcoma

Why and What

1. Osteochondroma with Malignant Transformation into Chondrosarcoma

In a pedunculated osteochondroma the cortex of the host bone and the cortex of the osteochondroma merge. In this case the peduncle does not show any cortex.

The minute punctate calcifications within the tumor prove that it is a chondroid lesion. The irregular, lobular shape with peripheral enhancement can be found in chondroid lesions, and the hypointensity on T1-weighted images is also consistent with chondroid tumors. The hypointensity on T2-weighted images is uncommon in mature, but common in immature chondroid lesions. A chondroid top – typical for osteochondromas – can be discerned.

There are some signs of aggressive behavior, indicated by the blurred borders of the peduncle, and of slow growth, indicated by expansion and thinning of the cortex and marginal calcification. The age of the patient fits the diagnosis of chondrosarcoma.

2. Periosteal Osteosarcoma

The configuration of the lesion (pedunculated) would be somewhat uncommon for a periosteal osteosarcoma. Periosteal sarcoma – one form of juxtacortical osteosarcoma – may have a lot of chondroid matrix with typical calcifications. It is also commonly found in the second decade of life, and not in the age group represented by our patient.

Final Diagnosis

Dedifferentiated Chondrosarcoma

Definition. An aggressive tumor develops, generally in a grade 1 or grade 2 central chondrosarcoma, and is histologically an osteosarcoma, fibrosarcoma, or malignant fibrous histiocytoma. Dedifferentiation can occur in either primary or secondary chondrosarcoma, and in recurrent low-grade chondrosarcoma.

Incidence. Dedifferentiation occurs in 10–15% of all central chondrosarcomas.

Age, sex distribution. There is a predilection for males, with a sex ratio of 1.5:1. Dedifferentiated chondrosarcomas are generally observed over the age of 50 years.

Location. Preferred sites are the pelvis, the femur, especially proximal, the proximal humerus, and the scapula.

Therapy. The treatment includes wide and radical surgical excision followed by chemotherapy.

Prognosis. Generally poor.

Remarks

The diagnosis of dedifferentiated chondrosarcoma is a histologic one. The tumor has one of the worst prognoses of all chondrosarcomas. Usually this lesion is based on a longstanding, low-grade cartilage tumor with remodeling expansion – as in our case – and a superimposed high-grade tumor. This clearly supports the theory that within a malignant chondroid tumor, there may be distinct cell clones with different degrees of differentiation.

Case 34   Lower Leg

History

This 24-year-old woman with type I diabetes mellitus had been on insulin therapy for 13 years.

Two months before hospital admission she sustained cramps and swelling in both lower legs for 1 day. She recovered almost completely, but swelling and pain remained in the left calf. Duplex sonography of the left calf gave rise to suspicion of a venous thrombosis, but could not be proven by phlebography. On clinical groups, thromboplebitis was assumed and treated. Because there was no clinical improvement, MRI was performed. Clinical examination at that time revealed a soft tissue tumor 7–10 cm in diameter within the gastrocnemius muscle. The patient could not straighten her left leg. The lower leg and foot were swollen.

Imaging

1. Plain Film Radiographs

Fig. 34.1
*Left lower leg,
a.p. projection*

No abnormalities are visualized within the tibia or fibula.

2. Magnetic Resonance Imaging

Fig. 34.2
Left lower leg

a T2-weighted image, axial plane
b T1-SE after contrast administration, axial plane
c T1-SE after contrast administration, sagittal plane

On axial T2-weighted images the medial head of the gastrocnemius muscle is diffusely enlarged and reveals abnormally high signal intensity with demarcation of irregularly formed hypointense zones in the medial aspects. The border with the intermuscular septum is blurred. After injection of contrast medium T1-SE images demonstrate enhancement of the whole medial part of the gastrocnemius muscle, the septum and the adjacent segment of the lateral gastrocnemius muscle. There are obvious nonenhancing necrotic areas centrally. Sagittal views outline the full extension of the lesion. The bony parts are not involved.

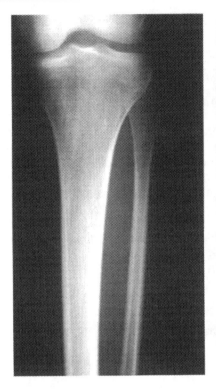

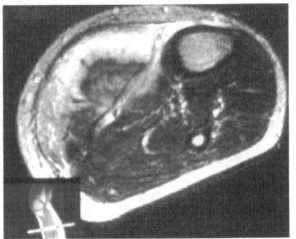

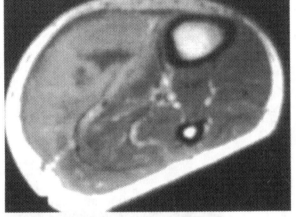

Fig. 34.1. Left lower leg, a. p. projection

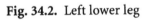

Fig. 34.2. Left lower leg

a T2-weighted image, axial plane
b T1-SE after contrast administration, axial plane
c T1-SE after contrast administration, sagittal plane

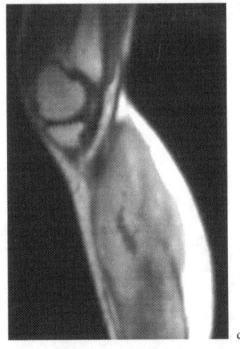

Differential Diagnosis Based on Radiographs

– No diagnosis could be postulated

Differential Diagnosis Based on Radiographs and Further Studies

– Myositis
– Malignant fibrous histiocytoma
– Rhabdomyosarcoma
– Fibromatosis

Why and What

1. Myositis
The diffuse nature of the lesion and its compartmental appearance might suggest a diffuse inflammatory process. There is also no evident mass effect, and central necroses can be observed in diffuse inflammatory processes. Myositis ossificans in an early phase is less probable. The typical zonal architecture of myositis ossificans, calcification at the rim, and central lucency can all be seen in such a case, probably owing to central necrosis and peripheral demarcation. There was no evidence of trauma and the patient did not inject insulin in the calf.

2. Malignant Fibrous Histiocytoma (of Soft Tissue)
Malignant fibrous histiocytoma is, next to liposarcoma, the most common malignant soft tissue tumor. It has a preferred localization in the lower limb (thigh) and retroperitoneum; however, it affects older age groups (50–70 years). The tumor replaces the normal structures and is a solid inhomogeneous mass. MFH cannot be completely ruled out, although the short history and the youth of the patient speak against this aggressive tumor. The blurred appearance and the invasion of the lateral head of the gastrocnemius muscle is one sign in favor of potential malignancy.

3. Rhabodmyosarcoma
Rhabdomyosarcoma is a tumor of the young (10–23 years). Radiographically it is an aggressive solid tumor. As in MFH, invasion of muscle is a sign of aggressiveness, which can be found in malignancy and inflammation, although in this case other typical signs such as solid masses and mass effect cannot be observed.

4. Fibromatosis (Desmoid Tumor)
This tumor grows very slowly over a number of years and has a compact and densely fibrous structure. These findings do not fit the observations in the present case.

Final Diagnosis

Unspecific Myositis with Vascular Lesions and Necrosis in Muscle Fibers

Inflammation of the muscle may occur in a variety of infectious disorders caused by viruses, bacteria, protozoa, and parasites. In this case the cause of the myositis remained unclear. The patient recovered completely within 3 months with conservative therapy. The (pseudo)inflammatory process was probably based on multiple microvascular occlusions leading to myositis. It can sometimes be very difficult to distinguish a soft tissue tumor from inflammation. In a questionable soft tissue mass the imaging method that should be used is MRI.

Case 35   Knee, Distal Femur

History

This 39-year-old man suffered from pain in the distal femur and knee joint. Palpation revealed no abnormality. No limitation of hip and knee movement was observed at the first clinical examination.

Imaging

1. Plain Film Radiographs

Fig. 35.1
Right knee and distal femur, lateral projection

A plain film radiograph of the knee reveals on the distal femur metaphysis an extraosseous lesion with a sclerotic rim measuring about 1 × 2 cm. In the lateral projection a cortical exostosis-like soft tissue calcification, 1.5 × 2 cm in size, with cortical irregularity on the dorsal side can be seen. The adjacent cortical and trabecular bone are without signs of destruction (Fig. 35.1).

2. Magnetic Resonance Imaging

Fig. 35.2
Right knee and distal femur

a STIR, coronal plane
b T1-SE, axial plane
c T1-SE after contrast administration, sagittal plane

MR images reveal a 3 × 4 cm, periosteal mass of the dorsal aspect of the distal femoral metaphyses (Fig. 35.2a). On T1-SE images there are foci of high signal intensity in the center of the lesion (Fig. 35.2b), with otherwise low signal intensity. Low and more marginal enhancement after Gd-DTPA administration can be seen (Fig. 35.2c). In connection with this lesion, the corticalis demonstrates signs of thinning. No infiltration of the muscles is demonstrated.

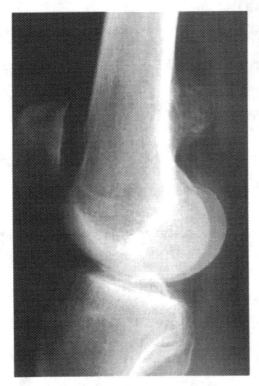

Fig. 35.1. Right knee and distal femur, lateral projection

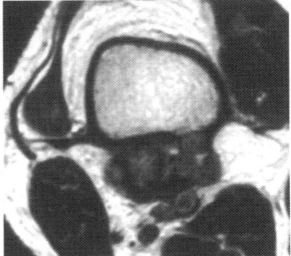

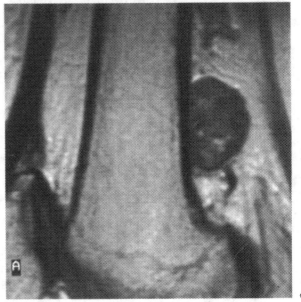

Fig. 35.2. Right knee and distal femur

a STIR, coronal plane
b T1-SE, axial plane
c T1-SE after contrast administration, sagittal plane

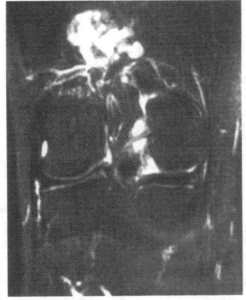

Why and What

Radiography reveals a small and incomplete cortical defect with a soft tissue calcification, whereas MRI demonstrates a small parosteal mass, suggesting a cartilaginous origin.

1. Parosteal Chondroma or Juxtacortical Chondroma

This is an uncommon lesion of bone. There is no gender predilection, and the age of the patients ranges from 4 to 70 years. The tumor occurs in the humerus, femur, and fingers, where the lesions are metaphyseal with the majority in the proximal metaphysis. The tumor appears to originate in the periosteum or cortex without evidence of medullary cavity involvement. Therefore the patient's age, the location, and the morphology of cortical bone and bone marrow confirm this diagnosis. Furthermore, of this lesion's signal characteristics with high intensity on T2-weighting and only marginal enhancement after administration of contrast medium suggest a cartilaginous mass. Central high signal intensities on T1-weighted images could represent fatty bone marrow, depenting on the bony structure or after calcification of cartilage.

2. Parosteal or Juxtacortical Chondrosarcoma

With this tumor the patients are older and the sarcomas tend to be larger. A more aggressive radiologic pattern with cortical destruction would be expected, which makes the diagnosis less probable in this case. However, there is some irregular cortical thickening and pronounced marginal contrast medium enhancement in our patient.

3. Osteochondroma

As an exostosis protrudes from the cortical surface its medullary and cortical bone is continuous with that of the underlying osseous structure, which could be clearly excluded in this case, especially by MRI.

4. Parosteal Osteosarcoma

This tumor features central ossifying foci with irregular outlines, and it may be connected to the underlying bone by a stalk. Parosteal osteosarcoma arises in the cortex of the metaphysis of a tubular bone and produces cortical thickening and spiculated osteoid matrix. Because of these signs this entity is very unlikely in this case, although the site is typical.

Final Diagnosis

Benign Parosteal Chondroma

Definition. Parosteal chondroma is a variety of chondroma that develops at the surface of the bone under the periosteum.

Synonym. Juxtacortical chondroma.

Age, sex distribution. Parosteal chondroma occurs from childhood to the fourth decade of life. There is a predilection for males, with a sex ratio of 2:1.

Location. Long bones, especially proximal humerus and fingers.

Therapy. En bloc excision, marginal or wide.

Prognosis. In the case of intralesional resection local recurrence can occur.

Case 36   Knee

History

This 52-year-old women experienced paresthesia and pain around the left knee. Pain increased at night. For years she had had varicosities on both lower legs. Hysterectomy had been carried out 8 years previously.

Imaging

1. Plain Film Radiographs

Fig. 36.1
Left knee, a. p. projection

Plain film radiographs show an irregular osteoblastic lesion in the left distal femur involving the lateral condyle. The cortical bone is partly destroyed and there is also an extracortical soft tissue tumor with calcifications. The center of the lesion is located metaphyseally with extension dia- and epiphyseally. The proximal tibia is not involved; the knee joint appears normal.

2. Computed Tomography

Fig. 36.2
Left knee, axial plane

Computed tomography demonstrates the cortex, which is partly irregular and partly destroyed or replaced by periostal spiculation or irregular new bone formation. There is also a calcified soft tissue mass dorsally and laterally. Laterally the border to the iliotibial tract and the lateral vastus muscle is faint or even indiscernible. There are some structural inhomogeneities in the surrounding subcutaneous soft tissue. There is no joint effusion.

3. Magnetic Resonance Imaging

Fig. 36.3
Left knee

a T1-SE, axial plane
b STIR, coronal plane
c T1-SE after contrast administration with fat suppression (SPIR), axial plane

MRI demonstrates the osteoblastic lesion in the distal femur laterally and dorsally. On the axial T1-weighted image the bright fatty marrow is replaced completely by low-intensity blastoma tissue (Fig. 36.3a). The calcified parts are also hypointense and therefore indistinguishable. On the T2-weighted inversion recovery image the solid tumor is moderately and inhomogeneously hyperintense (Fig. 36.3b). The cortex of the patella is preserved, but the tumor just touches the surface of the cortex. Above the patella the fluid-filled suprapatellar bursa is visualized. There is also a hyperintense line bordering the tumor next to the iliotibial tract and the lateral vastus muscle. Around the lateral condyle some effusion is outlined too. The tumor has direct contact with the body of the lateral meniscus. The collateral ligament is somewhat thickened and shows minute linear hypointensities (calcifications or fibrosis). After i.v. injection of contrast medium the whole tumor, except the calcifications, shows marked enhancement. The dorsal soft tissue touches the neurovascular bundle, but the fatty tissue in between seems to be preserved except in one slice. Caudally this soft tissue tumor reaches the cruciate ligaments. No infiltration can be documented, and no skip lesions are seen.

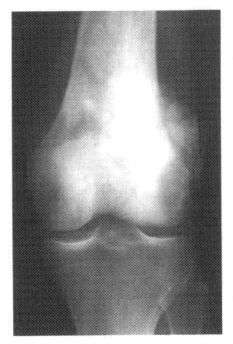

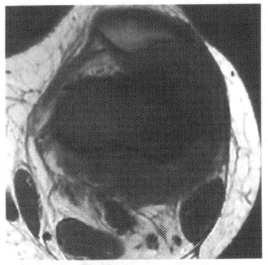

Fig. 36.1. Left knee, a. p. projection

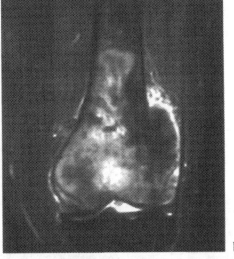

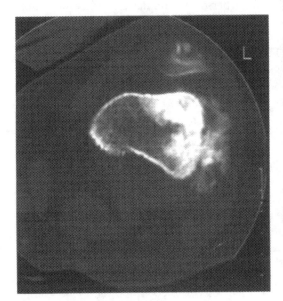

Fig. 36.2. Left knee, axial plane

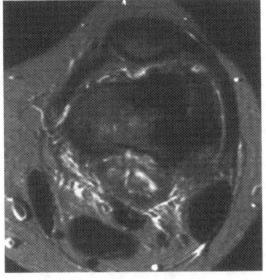

Fig. 36.3. Left knee

a T1-SE, axial plane
b STIR, coronal plane
c T1-SE after contrast administration with fat suppression (SPIR), axial plane

Differential Diagnosis Based on Radiographs

– Osteosarcoma

Differential Diagnosis Based on Radiographs and Further Studies

CT

– Conventional osteo-sarcoma
– Parosteal osteosarcoma (dedifferentiated, grade 3)

MRI

– Conventional (medullary) osteo-sarcoma
– Parosteal osteosarcoma

Why and What

1. Conventional (Medullary) Osteosarcoma

The lesion is an aggressive blastoma with cortical spiculation, cortical destruction, and infiltration of soft tissue, with calcification and new bone formation. There are no typical chondroid calcifications. Some 5–8% of all conventional osteosarcomas are found in the age group 40–70 years. The degree of radiopacity reflects a combination of the amounts of calcified matrix and osteoid produced by the tumor. Only 10% of conventional osteosarcomas are mainly osteosclerotic.

2. Parosteal Osteosarcoma

There are four different variants of juxtacortical osteosarcomas:

1. Parosteal (grade I) osteosarcoma
2. Dedifferentiated (grade II–III) parosteal osteosarcoma
3. Periosteal osteosarcoma
4. High-grade surface osteosarcoma

The four variants together account for about 7–8% of all osteosarcomas. Parosteal (grade I) sarcomas are slow-growing tumors with good prognosis. They are typically located at the posterior aspect of the distal femur. They demonstrate periosteal growth on the surface of the bone and can be located in the midshaft of a long bone. Most lesions occur in the second decade of life. The sparing of the medullary cavity for a long time is characteristic.

High-grade surface osteosarcomas represent less than 1% of all osteosarcomas. The radiologic features are the same as in periosteal and parosteal osteosarcoma. Histologically this tumor is difficult to distinguish from conventional osteosarcoma. Frequently the cortex and medullary cavity are involved.

Dedifferentiated parosteal osteosarcoma very often arises in a low-grade parosteal osteosarcoma. The lesion undergoes transformation to a high-grade malignancy. Radiographically it mimics a conventional parosteal osteosarcoma, but there is medullary and soft tissue invasion.

Final Diagnosis

Osteoblastic, Sclerosing Osteosarcoma (Grade 3)

Definition. Osteosarcoma is a neoplasm with proliferating malignant cells that produce osteoid matrix. Osteoid, chondroid or fibromatoid differentiation may be predominant.

Incidence. Except for myeloma, osteosarcoma is the most common primary bone tumor. Its incidence is about 4–6 cases per 1 million inhabitants per year.

Age, sex distribution. Seventy-five percent of all cases are manifested between 10 and 30 years of age. The peak incidence is the 2nd decade. There is a predilection for males, with a sex ratio of 1.5–2:1.

Location. The preferential sites are the metaphyses of long bones, especially the distal femur, proximal femur, proximal humerus, and proximal tibia.

Therapy. The treatment consists of chemotherapy and wide or radical surgical excision. Radiotherapy has largely been abandoned. After biopsy, preoperative chemotherapy is performed. Generally the definitive surgical procedure is carried out 10 weeks after the biopsy. After the surgery, adjuvant chemotherapy is carried out.

Prognosis. The survival rate with surgical treatment alone was 10–20%. Generally pulmonary metastases occurred within 1–2 years after amputation. Nowadays these figures have changed drastically. The 5-year survival rate after chemotherapy is approximately 60–70%. The response to chemotherapy is the single most important prognostic factor. When the tumor necrosis exceeds 90%, the outcome is good in more than 80% of the cases. Other factors influencing the prognosis are the size and the site of the tumor.

Remarks

The involvement of the cruciate ligaments and/or collateral ligaments has a great bearing on the surgical management.
Joint effusion is no proof of involvement, but an important hint. Radiographic calcification or noncalcification may not correspond to the histologic report of osteolytic or osteoblastic features.

Case 37   Lower Leg

History

This 58-year-old man had had paralysis of the left peroneus nerve since the age of 15. At that time – as far as he remembered – he had severe pain in his left lower limb after a soccer trauma.

He had now developed a quickly growing soft tissue mass (within 5–6 weeks) in the lower limb. At the time of palpation the tumor measured about 4 × 8 cm and was soft. There were no signs of inflammation.

Imaging

1. Plain Film Radiographs

Fig. 37.1
Left tibia and fibula

a A. p. projection
b Enlargement of the lesion

Plain film radiographs show several, irregularly formed, but well-defined calcifications within the anterior muscle space between the tibia and fibula. In the middle third a more homogeneous and somewhat less dense mass 8 cm in length and 2–3 cm in depth can be outlined. It corresponds to the palpable soft tissue mass.

2. Magnetic Resonance Imaging

Fig. 37.2
Left tibia and fibula

a T1-SE, sagittal plane
b T2-SE, coronal plane
c T1-SE after contrast administration, axial plane
d T1-SE after contrast administration, sagittal plane

There is a large, well-defined, inhomogeneous and on T1- and T2-weighted sequences hypointense mass between the tibia and fibula anteriorly. It covers a length of about 20 cm in craniocaudal extension (Figs. 37.2a, b).

After i.v. injection of contrast medium the surrounding soft tissue shows only little reactive enhancement, whereas the tumor remains hypointense (Figs. 37.2c, d).

On the axial views involvement of the anterior tibial muscle can be observed and there is also a close relation to the anterior vascular bundle with the peroneus nerve (Fig. 37.2c). The lateral cortex of the tibia is somewhat thinner; the fatty marrow is normal.

Both the thinning and the paucity of reactive signs indicate the process grows very slowly or not at all. The homogeneous, anteriorly expanding mass is the palpable soft tissue mass.

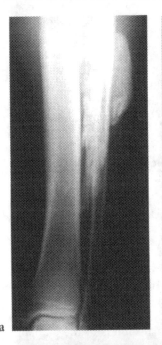
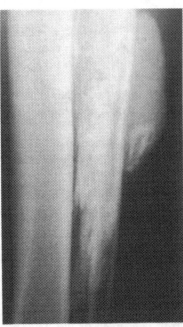

a

b

Fig. 37.1. Left tibia and fibula

a A.p. projection
b Enlargement of the lesion

◀

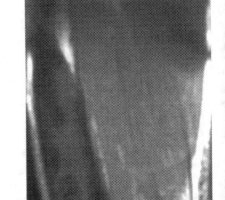

a, b

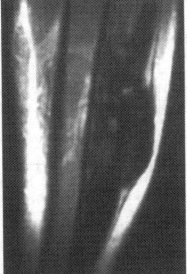

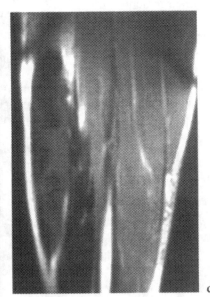

d

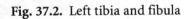

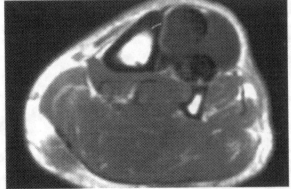

c

Fig. 37.2. Left tibia and fibula

a T1-SE, sagittal plane
b T2-SE, coronal plane
c T1-SE after contrast administration, axial plane
d T1-SE after contrast administration, sagittal plane

Differential Diagnosis Based on Radiographs

- Heterotopic ossification

Differential Diagnosis Based on Radiographs and Further Studies

- Regressive calcifications after trauma (operation)
- Regressive calcifications due to neural paralysis
- Tumor calcifications (osteosarcoma, chondrosarcoma; hemangioma, lipoma)
- Melorheostosis

Why and What

1. Regressive Calcifications After Trauma (Myositis Ossificans)
The history of the patient suggests a posttraumatic lesion, probably after bleeding, with calcification and cystic-necrotic changes which involve the peroneal nerve and parts of the tibialis anterior muscle. After years, for unknown reasons, reactive, inflammatory changes may have developed and led to the acute problem.
A lucent zone bordering the tibia (cleavage sign) can be observed. There are no signs of an aggressive tumor.
Zonal architecture, however, a characteristic sign, cannot be outlined.

2. Regressive Calcifications due to Neural Paralysis
In paraplegic patients involved muscles may calcify within months. In this case the peroneal nerve (pars profunda) paralysis would lead to calcifications within the extensor hallucis, extensor digiti and tibialis anterior muscles. However, in this case trauma was followed by paralysis.

3. Tumor Calcifications
Tumor calcifications can be found in benign and malignant lesions. However, this lesion does not reveal any aggressiveness. Benign tumors such as lipomas or hemangiomas, can be ruled out on the basis of the missing MRI characteristics. Moreover, no abnormal vascularity is obvious after i.v. injection of contrast medium.

4. Melorheostosis (Monostotic)
Melorheostosis is a cortical thickening resembling wax dripping down one side of a candle (flowing hyperostosis). Usually it exhibits both parosteal and endosteal involvement and extends into the articular end of the bone. None of these features are seen here.

Final Diagnosis

Pseudotumoral Muscular Posttraumatic Ectopic Ossification

Definition. Myositis ossificans is a benign heterotopic soft tissue ossification that may result from any of several different causes. Some 60–75% of patients with localized soft tissue ossifications relate a history of trauma. The spontaneous cases are termed pseudomalignant osseous tumor of soft tissue. Despite the name of the disease, some cases lack inflammation as well as muscle involvement.

Age, sex distribution. Myositis ossificans traumatica usually appears in adolescents or young adults.

Location. The sites where myositis ossificans occurs are areas susceptible to injury. The ectopic bone formation may lie longitudinally along the axis of the muscle and may also be attached to the bone.

Therapy. Usually the lesion remains untreated, unless there are functional restrictions. Otherwise surgical removal is indicated.

Prognosis. Even without treatment, most patients remain stable and without discomfort for their whole life. The prognosis after surgery is generally very good, and relief of pain can be expected in almost all cases.

Case 38   Knee

History

This 70-year-old patient felt a nodule in the hollow of the left knee for several months. The soft nodule seemed to grow very slowly. In the last few weeks before presentation, paresthesias and pain in the left lower leg developed. At the clinical examination a well-circumscribed nodule in the left hollow of the knee could be palpated. On palpation the patient reported some pain. Hypesthesia of the lower leg was observed.

Imaging

1. Plain Film Radiographs

Fig. 38.1
Left knee, lateral projection

There are no osseous abnormalities. The soft tissue mass in the hollow of the knee can be outlined. There is no calcification.

2. Magnetic Resonance Imaging

Fig. 38.2
Left knee

a T1-SE, sagittal plane
b T1-SE after contrast administration with fat suppression (SPIR), sagittal plane
c T1-SE after contrast administration with fat suppression (SPIR), axial plane

On T1-SE images the mass can be identified as a hypointense lesion dorso-laterally, adjacent to the lateral gastrocnemius muscle. The lesion's size is 2.8 × 2.5 × 2 cm (Fig. 38.2a).

On T2-weighted images the lesion is centrally rather hypointense and surrounded by a hyperintense rim. After administration of contrast medium the lesion exhibits rather homogeneous enhancement.

The adjacent muscles are indented, but not infiltrated. Osseous structures are not involved. There is no connection with the joint space.

In the subchondral region of the patella and condyle there are several edematous regions (2–5 mm in size) which also show significant enhancement.

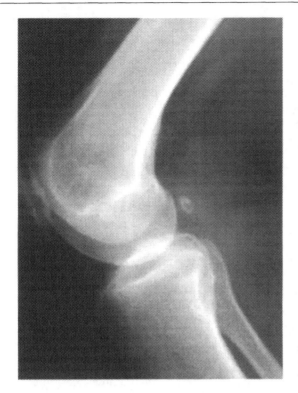

Fig. 38.1. Left knee, lateral projection

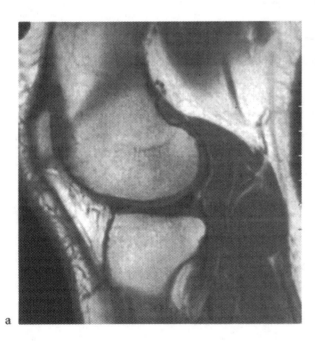

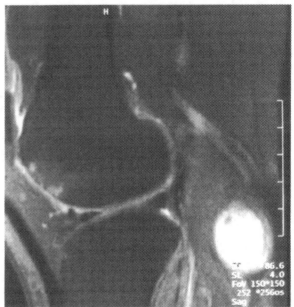

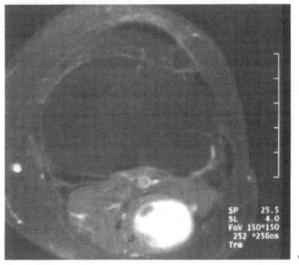

Fig. 38.2. Left knee

a T1-SE, sagittal plane
b T1-SE after contrast administration with fat suppression (SPIR), sagittal plane
c T1-SE after contrast administration with fat suppression (SPIR), axial plane

Why and What

1. Schwannoma

Peripheral neurinomas, in most cases deriving from the Schwann cells of the epi-, peri- or endoneurium are well encapsulated, and very rarely calcify. They may show areas of myxoid or cystic degeneration. They are hypointense on T1-weighted images, moderately hyperintense on T2-weighted images, and demonstrate significant contrast enhancement. In our case the lesion fulfills all clinical and radiological criteria of a schwannoma.

2. Hemangioma

Hemangioma are, besides lipoma, the most common benign soft tissue tumor. They reveal areas of irregular intermediate signal intensities that correspond with the vascular components. The remainder of the tumor remains hypointense or isointense, depending on the stage of possible bleedings. After injection of contrast medium delayed enhancement may be observed. Hemangiomas may also show calcification. These features are not demonstrated in our case.

3. Fibroma

Fibromas are fibrous lesions with hypointensity on T1- and T2-weighted images and have variable contrast enhancement, depending on the amount of fibrous tissue. Although the MRI findings are not really characteristic for a fibroma in our case, we cannot exclude this diagnosis.

Final Diagnosis

Schwannoma

Definition. This tumor is an encapsulated nerve sheath tumor consisting of two components, a highly ordered cellular component and a loose myxoid component.

Synonyms. Neurilemoma, benign neurinoma.

Symptoms. When it is located in a peripheral nerve, palpation reveals a tumor mass which is sharply painful, particularly with pressure. This sharp radiating pain is often accompanied by paresthesia. Deep-seated schwannomas are symptomatic because of their larger size and impingement on neighboring structures (compression of nerve roots, of the cauda equina or of the spinal cord in the more cranial sites).

Age, sex distribution. The tumor occurs at all ages, mainly between 20 and 50 years of age. There is no gender predilection.

Location. Schwannomas are most commonly located in the spinal roots, in the nerves of the mediastinum and of the retroperitoneum. In the periphery they are found on the flexor surfaces of the upper and lower extremities. Therefore, the peroneal and ulnar nerves are most often affected. Schwannomas almost always occur as solitary lesions, but in unusual instances, or in the setting of Recklinghausen's disease, multiple schwannomas may occur.

Therapy. Simple excision is not followed by recurrence.

Prognosis. Malignant transformation is exceedingly rare. After complete excision no local recurrence is observed.

Case 39   Knee

History

This 16-year-old boy presented with a history of nonspecific symptoms and signs, including pain, swelling and tenderness in the area of the medial left knee, for several months. Otherwise clinical evaluation and blood tests showed no abnormality.

Imaging

1. Plain Film Radiographs

Fig. 39.1
Left knee, lateral projection

At first glance the radiographs of the left knee joint seem to be normal. On closer inspection, however, a small and discrete osteolytic lesion with a diameter of 1 cm and a thin sclerotic rim can be seen in the lateral view (Fig. 39.1). The lesion is located eccentrically in the epiphysis of the proximal tibia. No foci of calcification are seen within the lesion. No soft tissue masses or pathologic fractures are obvious.

2. Magnetic Resonance Imaging

Fig. 39.2
Left knee

a T1-weighted image, sagittal plane
b T2-weighted GE image, (cartilage flash), coronal plane
c T2-weighted GE image, sagittal plane

Magnetic resonance imaging clearly demonstrates the lesion in an eccentric location in the dorsomedial aspect of the proximal epiphysis of the left tibia. The diameter is 10 mm. Signal is of low intensity in T1-weighted SE images (Fig. 39.2a), intermediate in the T1-weighted GE images (Fig. 39.2b), and intermediate to high in the T2-weighted GE images (Fig. 39.2c). The growing endplate is still present and is in contact with the lesion; however, no destruction of the end plate is evident.

A subtle rim around the lesion with hypointense signal can be discerned in all sequences. Further subtle diffuse signal alterations, hypointense on T1- and hyperintense on T2-weighted images, indicate moderate bone marrow edema.

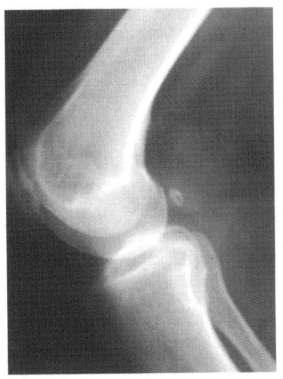

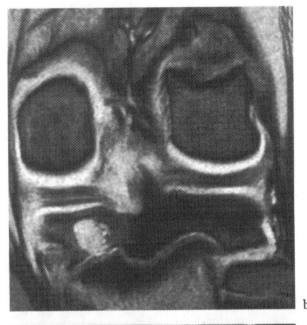

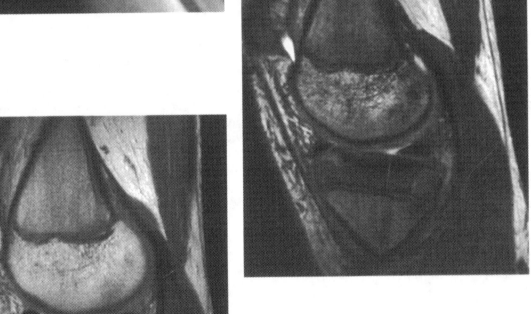

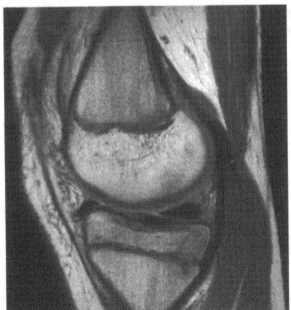

Why and What

1. Chondroblastoma

Chondroblastomas are most frequent in the second and third decades of life. Chondroblastomas generally arise in the epiphysis or apophysis of a long tubular bone. The femur, the humerus, and the tibia, as in this case, are the most frequent sites.

The radiographic features are characteristic: an osteolytic lesion, usually less than 5 cm in diameter, well defined and spheroid or oval in shape. A thin sclerotic rim may separate the tumor from the adjacent normal bone. Calcifications within the lesion are seen in 30–50% of patients. Soft tissue masses and pathologic fractures are rare.

Chondroblastomas are of variable signal intensity on T2-weighted SE MRI. However, generally high signal intensities which may come close to the signal of cartilage are observed, as in this case. Therefore the radiological appearance of the lesion is compatible with this diagnosis.

A possible absence of high signal intensity on T2-weighted images in some chondroblastomas may relate to a prominent cellular stroma and differs from the high signal intensity characteristic of hyaline cartilage, which is present in enchondromas, osteochondromas, and well-differentiated chondrosarcomas.

2. Intraosseous Ganglion

The location, size, and border as seen on plain film radiographs and the subtle surrounding bone marrow edema as evident on MRI would fit this diagnosis. However, other MRI findings – absence of a connecting duct between the knee joint and the lesion and lack of fluid-like signal intensity of the lesion – speak against an intraosseous ganglion. Usually perifocal bone marrow edema is absent.

3. Giant-Cell Tumor

The epiphyseal location is typical for this entity, but in the case of giant-cell tumor we would expect a higher age of the patient and, particularly, more aggressive behavior by the lesion.

4. Brodie's Abscess

Signs of abscess such as an inflammatory zoning of the lesion itself and a more pronounced perifocal reaction are not present in this case.

Final Diagnosis

Chondroblastoma

Definition. Benign tumor, involving of the epiphyseal or apophyseal region of the bone. Usually it manifests during late childhood or adolescence and is composed of cells considered to be chondroblasts.

Incidence. Chondroblastoma is an infrequent tumor.

Age, sex distribution. The tumor manifests most frequently in the second decade, but it can be found at any time of life. There is a predilection for males (3:1).

Location. The typical location is the epiphysis or apophysis in the growth cartilage. The sites most frequently affected are the epiphysis and apophysis of long bones, especially the humerus, femur and tibia. Less frequent locations are pelvis, scapula, talus, and calcaneus.

Therapy. Therapy usually consists of intralesional excision, additionally a few millimeters of the deep bony wall are removed and the bony wall is treated with phenol. The cavity is then filled with bone chips or other autologous grafts. In rare cases osteochondral bone allografts are used.

Recommended Reading

Osteoma

Greenspan A. Benign bone-forming lesions: osteoma, osteoid osteoma, and osteoblastoma. Skeletal Radiol 1993; 22: 485–500.

Lichtenstein L, Sawyer WR. Benign osteoblastoma: further observations and report of twenty additional cases. J Bone Joint Surg 1964; 46A: 755–765.

Sundaram M, Falbo S, McDonald D, Janney C. Surface osteomas of the appendicular skeleton. Am J Roentgenol 1996; 167: 1529–1533.

Osteoidosteoma

Assoun J, Richardi G, Railhac JJ, Baunin C, Fajadet P, Giron J, Maquin P, Haddad J, Bonnevialle P. Osteoid osteoma: MR imaging versus CT. Radiology 1994; 191: 217–223.

Cohen MD, Harrington TM, Ginsburg WW. Osteoid osteoma: 95 cases and a review of the literature. Semin Arthritis Rheum 1983; 12: 265–281.

Glass RB, Poznanski AR, Fisher MR, Shkolnik A, Dias L. MR imaging of osteoid osteoma. J Comput Tomogr 1986; 10: 1065–1067.

Klein MH, Shankman S. Osteoid osteoma: radiologic and pathologic correlation. Skeletal Radiol 1992; 21: 23–31.

Smith FW, Gilday DL, Scintigraphic appearances of osteoid osteoma. Radiology 1980; 137: 191–195.

Woods ER, Martel W, Mandell SH, Crabbe JP. Reactive soft-tissue mass associated with osteoid osteoma: correlation of MR imaging features with pathologic findings. Radiology 1993; 186: 221–225.

Youssef BA, Haddad MC, Zahrani A, Sharif HS, MorganJL, AI-Shahed M, AI Sabty A, Choudary R. Osteoid ostoma and osteoblastoma: MRI appearances and the significance of ring enhancement. Eur Radiol 1996; 6: 291–296.

Osteoblastoma

Azouz EM, Kozlowski K, Marton D, Sprague P, Zerhouni A, Assalah F. Osteoid osteoma and osteoblastoma of the spine in children. Report of 22 cases with brief literature review. Pediatr Radio 1986; 16: 25–31.

Della Rocca C, Huvus AG. Osteoblastoma: varied histological presentations with a benign clinical course – 55 cases. Am J Surg Pathol 1996; 20: 841–850.

Kroon HM, Schurmans J. Osteoblastoma: clinical and radiologic findings in 98 new cases. Radiology 1990; 175: 783–790.

Osteosarcoma

Kumar N, David R, Madewell JE, Lindell MM Jr. Radiographic spectrum of osteogenic sarcoma. Am J Roentgenol 1987; 148: 767–772.

Moore TE, King AR, Kathol MH, El-Khoury GY, Palmer R, Downey PR. Sarcoma in Paget disease of bone: clinical, radiologic, and pathologic features in 22 cases. Am J Roentgenol 1991; 156: 1199–1203.

Norton KI, Hermann G. Abdelwahab IF, Klein MJ, Granowetter LF, Rabinowitz JG. Epiphyseal involvement in osteosarcoma. Radiology 1991; 180: 813–816.

Onikul E, Fletcher BD, Parham DM, Chen G. Accuracy of MR imaging for estimating intraosseous extent of osteosarcoma. Am J Roentgenol 1996; 167: 1211–1215.

Rosenberg ZS, Leu S, Schmahmann S, Steiner GC, Beltran J, Present D. Osteosarcoma: subtle, rare, and misleading plain film features. Am J Roentgenol 1995; 165: 1209–1214.

Enchondroma, Periosteal Chondroma, Enchondromatoses, Soft Tissue Chondroma

Bansal M, Goldman AB, DiCarlo HF, McCormack R. Soft tissue chondromas: diagnosis and differential diagnosis. Skeletal Radiol 1993; 22: 309–315.

Boriani S, Bacchini P, Bertoni F, Campanacci M. Periosteal chondroma. A review of twenty cases. J Bone Joint Surg 1983; 65A: 205–212.

Moser RP, Gilkey FW, Madewell JF. Enchondroma. In: Moser RP, ed. Cartilaginous tumors of the skeleton. AFIP atlas of radiologic-pathologic correlation, vol 2. Philadelphia: Hanley and Belfus, 1990; 8–34.

Ragsdale BD, Sweet DE, Vinh TN. Radiology as gross pathology in evaluating chondroid tumors. Hum Pathol 1989; 20: 930-951.

Osteochondroma, Multiple Hereditary Osteochondromatoses

Cohen EK, Kressel HY, Frank TS, Fallon M, Burk DL Jr, Dalinka MK, Schiebler ML. Hyaline cartilage-origin bone and soft-tissue neoplasms: MR appearance and histologic correlation. Radiology 1988; 167: 477–481.

Fairbank TJ. Dysplasia epiphysealis hemimelica (tarso-epiphyseal aclasis). J Bone Joint Surg 1956; 38 Br: 237-257.

Geirnaerdt MJA, Bloem JL, Eulderink F, Hogendoorn PCW, Taminiau AH. Cartilaginous tumors: correlation of gadolinium-enhanced MR imaging and histopathologic findings. Radiology 1993; 186: 813–817.

Hudson TM, Springfield DS, Spanier SS, Enneking WF, Hamlin DJ. Benign exostoses and exostotic chondrosarcomas: evaluation of cartilage thickness by CT. Radiology 1984; 152: 595-599.

Chondroblastoma

Braunstein F, Martel W, Weatherbee L. Periosteal bone apposition in chondroblastoma. Skeletal Radiol 1979; 4: 34-36.

Cohen EK, Kressel HY, Frank TS, Fallon M, Burk DL Jr, Dalinka MK, Schiebler ML. Hyaline cartilage-origin bone and soft-tissue neoplasms: MR appearance and histologic correlation. Radiology 1988; 167: 477–481.

Gardner DJ, Azouz EM. Solitary lucent epiphyseal lesions in children. Skeletal Radiol 1988; 17: 497-504.

Hayes CW, Conway WF, Sundaram M. Misleading aggressive MR imaging: appearance of some benign musculoskeletal lesions. Radiographics 1992; 12: 1119-1134.

Kroon HM, Bloem JL, Holscher HC, van der Woude HJ, Reijnierse M, Taminiau AHM. MR imaging of edema accompanying benign and malignant bone tumors. Skeletal Radiol 1994; 23: 261-269.

Weatherall PT, Maale GE, Mendelsohn DB, Sherry CS, Erdman WE, Pascoe HR. Chondroblastoma: classic and confusing appearance at MR imaging. Radiology 1994; 190: 467–474.

Yamamura S, Sato K, Sugiura H. Iwata H. Inflammatory reaction in chondroblastoma. Skeletal Radiol 1996; 25: 371–376.

Chondromyxoid Fibroma

Feldman F, Hecht HL, Johnston AD. Chondromyxoid fibroma of bone. Radiology 1970; 94: 249–260.

White PG, Saunders L, Orr W, Friedman L. Chondromyxoid fibroma. Skeletal Radiol 1996; 25: 79–81.

Wilson AJ. Kyriakos M, Ackerman LV. Chondromyxoid fibroma: Radiographic appearance in 38 cases and in a review of the literature. Radiology 1991; 179: 513-518. Also Erratum. Radiology 1991; 180: 586.

Chondrosarcoma

Amir U, Amir G, Mogle P, Pogrund H. Extraskeletal soft tissue chondrosarcoma. Case report and review of the literature. Clin Orthop 1985; 198: 219–223.

Aoki JA, Sone S, Fujioka F, Terajama K, Ishii K, Karakida O, lmai S, Sakai F, Imai Y. MR of enchondroma and chondrosarcoma: rings and arcs of Gd-DTPA enhancement. J Comput Assist Tomogr 1991; 15: 1011–1016.

Brien LW, Mirra JM, Herr R. Benign and malignant cartilage tumors of bone and joints: their anatomic and theoretical basis with an emphasis on radiology, pathology, and clinical biology. Skeletal Radiol 1997; 26: 325–353.

Crim JR, Seeger LL. Diagnosis of low-grade chondrosarcoma. Radiology 1993; 189: 503–504.

De Beuckeleer LHL, De Schepper AMA, Ramon F. Magnetic resonance imaging of cartilaginous tumors: is it useful or necessary? Skeletal Radiol 1996; 25: 137–141.

Mercuri M, Picci P, Campanacci M, Rulli E. Dedifferentiated chondrosarcoma. Skeletal Radiol 1995; 24: 409–416.

Rosenthal DJ, Schiller AL, Mankin HJ. Chondrosarcoma: correlation of radiological and histological grade. Radiology 1984; 150: 21–26.

Fibribrotic Cortical Defect and Nonossifying Fibroma

Kumar R, Madewell JE, Lindell MM, Swischuk LB. Fibrous lesions of bones. Radiographics 1990; 10: 237–256.

Ritschl P, Karnel F, Hajek PC. Fibrous metaphyseal defects - determination of their origin and natural history using a radiomorphological study. Skeletal Radiol 1988; 17: 8–15.

Ritschl P, Hajek PC, Pechmann U. Fibrous metaphyseal defects. Magnetic resonance imaging appearances. Skeletal Radiol 1989; 18: 253–259.

Benign Fibrous Histiocytoma

Clarke BE, Xipell JM, Thomas DR. Benign fibrous histiocytoma of bone. Am J

Hamada T, Ito H, Araki Y, Fujii K, lnoue M, Ishida O. Benign fibrous histio-
    cytoma of the femur: review of three cases. Skeletal Radiol 1996; 25: 25–29.

Periosteal Desmoid

Pennes DR, Braunstein EM, Glazer GM. Computed tomography of cortical
    desmoid. Skeletal Radiol 1984; 12: 40–42.
Resnick D, Greenway G. Distal femoral cortical defects, irregularities, and ex-
    cavations: a critical review of the literature with the addition of histologic
    and paleopathologic data. Radiology 1982; 143: 345–354.

Fibrous Dysplasia

Daffner RH, Rirks DR, Gehweiler JA Jr, Heaston DK. Computed tomography
    of fibrous dysplasia. Am J Roentgenol 1982; 139: 943–948.
Jee WH, Choi KH, Choe BY, Park JM, Shiin KS. Fibrous dysplasia: MR imaging
    characteristics with radiopathologic correlation. Am J Roentgenol 1996;
    167: 1523–1527.
Utz JA, Kransdorf MJ, Jelinek JS, Moser RP, Berrey BH. MR appearance of
    fibrous dysplasia. J Comput Assist Tomogr 1989; 13: 845–851.

Osteofibrous Dysplasia

Campanacci M, Laus M. Osteofibrous dysplasia of the tibia and fibula. J Bone
    Joint Surg 1981; 63A: 367–375.
Czerniak B, Rojas-Corona RR, Dorfman HD. Morphologic diversity of long bone
    adamantinoma. The concept of differentiated (regressing) adamantinoma
    and its relationship to osteofibrous dysplasia. Cancer 1989; 64: 2319–2334.
Zeanah WR, Hudson TM, Springfield DS. Computed tomography of ossifying
    fibroma of the tibia. J Comput Assist Tomogr 1983; 7: 688–691.

Desmoplastic Fibroma

Crim JR, Gold RH, Mirra JM, Eckardt JJ, Bassett LW. Desmoplastic fibroma of
    bone: radiographic analysis. Radiology 1989; 172: 827–832.
Gebhardt MC, Campbell CJ, Schiller AL, Mankin HJ. Desmoplastic fibroma of
    bone. A report of eight cases and review of the literature. J Bone Joint Surg
    1985; 67A: 732–747.
Taconis WK, Schotte HE, van der Heul RO. Desmoplastic fibroma of bone: a
    report of 18 cases. Skeletal Radiol 1994; 23: 283–288.

Fibrosarcoma und Malignant Fibrous Histiocytoma

Aisen AM, Martel W, Braunstein EM, McMillin KI, Phillips WA, Kling TF.
    MRI and CT evaluation of primary bone and soft-tissue tumors. Am J
    Roentgenol 1986; 146: 749–756.
Bloem JL, Taminiau AH, Eulderink F, Hermans J, Pauwels EK. Radiologic stag-
    ing of primary bone sarcoma: MR imaging, scintigraphy, angiography, and
    CT correlated with pathologic examination. Radiology 1988; 169: 805–810.

Murphey MD, Gross TM, Rosenthal HG. Musculoskeletal malignant fibrous histiocytoma: radiologic-pathologic correlation. Radiographics 1994; 14: 807–826.

Ros PR, Viamonte M Jr, Rywlin AM. Malignant fibrous histiocytoma: mesenchymal tumor of ubiquitous origin. Am J Roentgenol 1984; 142: 753–759.

Langerhans-Cell Granuloma (Eosinophilic Granuloma)

Beltran J, Aparisi F, Marti Bonmati L, Rosenberg ZS, Present D, Steiner GS. Eosinophilic granuloma: MRI manifestations. Skeletal Radiol 1993; 22: 157–161.

David R, Oria RA, Kumar R, Singelton EB, Lindell MM, Shirkhoda A, Madewell JF. Radiologic features of eosinophilic granuloma of bone. Am J Roentgenol 1989; 153: 1021–1026.

De Schepper AM, Ramon F, Van Marck E. MR imaging of eosinophilic granuloma: report of 11 cases. Skeletal Radiol 1993; 22: 163–166.

Meyer JS, Harty MP, Mahboubi S, Heyman S. Zimmerman RA, Womer RB, Dormans JP, Anglo GJ. Langerhans cells histiocytosis: presentation and evolution of radiologic findings with clinical correlation. Radiographics 1995; 15: 1135–1146.

Ewing Sarcoma

Cavazzana AO, Miser JS, Jefferson J, Triche TJ. Experimental evidence for a neural origin of Ewing's sarcoma of bone. Am J Parhol 1987; 127: 507–518.

Coombs RJ, Zeiss J, McKann K, Phillips E. Multifocal Ewing's tumor of the skeletal system. Skeletal Radiol 1986; 15: 254–257.

Estes DN, Magill HL, Thompson EL, Hayes FA. Primary Ewing sarcoma: follow-up with Ga-67 scintigraphy. Radiology 1990; 177: 449–453.

Friedman B, Hanoaka H. Round cell sarcoma of hone. J Bone Joint Surg 1971; 53A: 1118–1136.

Frouge C, Vanel D, Coffre C, Couanet D, Contesso G, Sarrazin D. The role of magnetic resonance imaging in the evaluation of Ewing's sarcoma. A report of 27 cases. Skeletal Radiol 1988; 17: 387–392.

Levine F, Levine C. Ewing tumor of rib: radiologic findings and computed tomography contribution. Skeletal Radiol 1983; 9: 227–233.

Vanel D, Contesso G, Couanet D, Piekarski JD, Sarrazin D, Masselot J. Computed tomography in the evaluation of 4l cases of Ewing's sarcoma. Skeletal Radiol 1982; 9: 8–13.

Malignant Lymphoma

Beackley MC, Lau BP, Ring ER. Bone involvement in Hodgkin's disease. Am J Roentgenol 1972; 114: 559–563.

Bragg DG, Colby TV, Ward JH. New concepts in the non-Hodgkin lymphomas: radiologic implications. Radiology 1986; 159: 289–304.

Daffner RN, Lupetin AR, Dash N, Deeb ZL, Sefczek RJ, Shapiro RL. MRI in the detection of malignant infiltration of bone marrow. Am J Roentgenol 1986; 146: 353–358.

Fishman EK, Kuhlman JE, Jones RJ. CT of lymphoma: spectrum of disease. Radiographics 1991; 11: 647–669.

Malloy PC, Fishman EK, Magid D. Lymphoma of bone, muscle, and skin: CT findings. Am J Roentgenol 1992; 159: 805–809.

Resnick D, Haghighi P. Myeloproliferative disorders. In: Resnick D, ed. Bone and joint imaging. Philadelphia: WB Saunders, 1989; 703–714.

Stiglbauer R, Augustin I, Kramer J, Schurawitzki H, Imbof H, Rodaszkiewicz T. MR in the diagnosis of primary lymphoma of bone: correlation with histopathology. J Comput Assist Tomogr 1992; 16: 248–253.

Multiple Myeloma (Plasmacytoma, Kahler Disease)

Fruehwald FX, Tscholakoff D, Schwaighofer B, Wicke L, Neuhold A, Ludwig H, Hajek PC. Magnetic resonance imaging of the lower vertebral column in patients with multiple myeloma. Invest Radiol 1988; 23: 193–199.

Lipshitz HI, Maithouse SR, Cunningham D, MacVicar AD, Husband JE. Multiple myeloma: appearance at MR imaging. Radiology 1992; 182: 833–837.

Meyer JE, Schulz MD. Solitary myeloma of bone: a review of 12 cases. Cancer 1974; 34: 438–440.

Resnick D, Haghighi P, Guerra J Jr. Bone sclerosis and proliferation in a man with multisystem disease. Invest Radiol 1984; 19: 1–6.

Stäbler A, Baur A, Bartl R, Munker R, Lamerz R, Reiser MF. Contrast enhancement and quantitative signal analysis in MR imaging of multiple myeloma: assessment of focal and diffuse growth patterns in marrow correlated with biopsies and survival rates. Am J Roentgenol 1996; 167: 1029–1036.

Woolfenden JM, Pitt MJ, Dune BCM, Moon TE. Comparison of bone scintigraphy and radiography in multiple myeloma. Radiology 1980; 134: 723–728.

Intraosseous Hemangioma, Cystic Angiomatoses, Lymphangioma, and Lymphangiomatoses

Boyle WJ. Cystic angiomatosis of bone. J Bone Joint Surg 1972; 54B: 626–636.

Cohen JW, Weinreb JC, Redman HC. Arteriovenous malformations of the extremities: MR imaging. Radiology 1986; 158: 475–479.

Friedman DP. Symptomatic vertebral hemangiomas: MR findings. Am J Roentgenol 1996; 167: 359–364.

Graham DY, Gonzales J, Kothari SM. Diffuse skeletal angiomatosis. Skeletal Radiol 1978; 3: 131–135.

Hawnaur JM, Whitehouse RW, Jenkins JPR, Isherwood I. Musculoskeletal haemangiomas: comparison of MRI with CT. Skeletal Radiol 1990; 19: 251–258.

Meyer JS, Hoffer FA, Barnes PD, Mulliken JB. Biological classification of soft-tissue vascular anomalies: MR correlation. Am J Roentgenol 1991; 157: 559–564.

Suh JS, Hwang C, Hahn SB. Soft tissue hemangiomas: MR manifestations in 23 patients. Skeletal Radiol 1994; 23: 621–625.

Hemangioendothelioma, Angiosarcoma, and Hemangiopericytoma

Abrahams TC, Bula W, Jones M. Epithelinoid hemangioendothelioma of bone. Skeletal Radiol 1992; 21: 509–513.

Alpern MB, Thorsen MK, Kellman GM, Pojunas K, Lawson TL. CT appearance of hemangiopericytoma. J Comput Assist Tomogr 1986; 10: 264–267.

Boutin RD, Spaeth HJ, Mangalik A, Sell JJ. Epitheloid hemangioendothelioma of bone. Skeletal Radiol 1996; 25: 391–395.

Campanacci M, Boriani S, Ciunti A. Hemangioendothelioma of bone: a study of 29 cases. Cancer 1980; 46: 804–814.

Lorigan JC, David CL, Evans HL, Wallace S. The clinical and radiologic manifestations of hemangiopericytoma. Am J Roentgenol 1989; 153: 345–349.

Steinbach LS, Ominsky SH, Shpall S, Perkocha LA. MR imaging of spindle cell hemangioendothelioma. J Comput Assist Tomogr 1991; 15: 155–157.

Giant-Cell Tumor

Aoki J, Tanikawa H, Ishii K, Seo GS, Kurakida O, Sone S, Ichikawa T, Kachi K. MR findings indicative of hemosiderin in giant-cell tumor of bone: frequency, cause, and diagnostic significance. Am J Roentgenol 1996; 166: 145–148.

Campanacci M, Baldini N, Boriani S, Sudanese A. Giant cell tumor of bone. J Bone Joint Surg 1987; 69A: 106–114.

Dahlin DC. Giant cell tumor of bone: Highlights of 407 cases. Am J Roentgenol 1985; 144: 955–960.

deSantos LA, Murray JA. Evaluation of giant cell tumor by computerized tomography. Skeletal Radiol 1978; 2: 205–212.

Herman SD, Mesgarzadeh M, Bonakdarpour A, Dalinka MK. The role of magnetic resonance imaging in giant cell tumor of bone. Skeletal Radiol 1987; 16: 635–643.

Maloney WJ, Vaughan LM, Jones HH, Ross J, Nagel DA. Benign metastasizing giant-cell tumor of bone. Report of three cases and review of the literature. Clin Orthop 1989; 243: 208–215.

May DA, Good RB, Smith DK, Parsons TW. MR imaging of musculoskeletal tumors and tumor mimickers with intravenous gadolinium: experience with 242 patients. Skeletal Radiol 1997; 26: 2–15.

Simple Bone Cyst

Cohen J. Etiology of simple bone cyst. J Bone Joint Surg 1970; 52A: 1493–1497.

Hertzanu Y, Mendelsohn DB, Gottschalk F. Aneurysmal bone cyst of the calcaneus. Radiology 1984; 151: 51–52.

Struhl S, Edelson C, Pritzker H, Seimon LP, Dorfman HD. Solitary (unicameral) bone cyst. The fallen fragment sign revisited. Skeletal Radiol 1989; 18: 261–265.

Aneurysmal Bone Cyst

Beltran J, Simon DC, Levy M, Herman L, Weis L, Mueller CF. Aneurysmal bone cysts: MR imaging at 1.5 T. Radiology 1986; 158: 689–690.

Bonakdarpour A, Levy WM, Aegerter F. Primary and secondary aneurysmal bone cysts: a radiological study of 75 cases. Radiology 1978; 126: 75–83.

Hudson TM. Fluid levels in aneurysmal bone cysts: a CT feature. Am J Roentgenol 1984; 141: 1001–1004.

Hudson TM. Scintigraphy of aneurysmal bone cysts. Am J Roentgenol 1984; 142: 761–765.

Kransdorf MJ, Sweet DE. Aneurysmal bone cyst: concept, controversy, clinical presentation, and imaging. Am J Roentgenol 1995; 164: 573–580.

Munk PL, Helms CA, Holt RG, Johnston J, Steinbach L, Neumann C. MR imaging of aneurysmal bone cysts. Am J Roentgenol 1989; 153: 99–101.

Zimmer WD, Berquist TH, McLeod RA, Sim FH, Pritchard DJ, Shives TC, Wold LE, May GR. Bone tumors: magnetic resonance imaging versus computed tomography. Radiology 1985; 155: 709–718.

Intraosseous Lipoma

Blacksin MF, Ende N, Benevenia J. Magnetic resonance imaging of intraosseous lipomas: a radiologic-pathologic correlation. Skeletal Radiol 1995; 24: 37–41.

Dooms GC, Hricak H, Sollitto RA, Higgins CB. Lipomatous tumors and tumors with fatty component: MR imaging potential and comparison of MR and CT results. Radiology 1985; 157: 479–483.

Levin ME, Vellet AD, Munk PL, McLean CA. lntraosseous lipoma of the distal femur: MRI appearance. Skeletal Radiol 1996; 25: 82–4.

Milgram JW. lntraosseous lipoma: Radiologic and pathologic manifestations. Radiology 1988; 167: 155–160.

Ramos A, Castello J, Sartoris DJ, Greenway GD, Resnick D, Haghighi P. Osseous lipoma: CT appearance. Radiology 1985; 157: 615–619.

Adamantinoma

Huvos AG, Marcove RC. Adamantinoma of long bones: a clinicopathological study of fourteen cases with vascular origin suggested. J Bone Joint Surg 1975; 57: 148–154.

Ishida T, Iijima T, Kikuchi F, Kitagawa T, Tanida T, Imamura T, Machinami R. A clinicopathological and immunohistochemical study of osteofibrous dysplasia, differentiated adamantinoma, and adamantinoma of long bones. Skeletal Radiol 1992; 21: 493–502.

Zehr RJ, Recht MP, Bauer TW. Adamantinoma. Skeletal Radiol 1995; 24: 553–555.

Chordoma

Meyer JE, Lepke RA, Lindfors KK, Pagani JJ, Hitschy JC, Hayman LA, Momose KJ, McGinnis B. Chordomas: their CT appearance in the cervical, thoracic and lumbar spine. Radiology 1984; 153: 693–696.

Rosenthal Dl, Scott JA, Mankin HJ, Wismet GL, Brady TJ. Sacrococcygeal chordoma: magnetic resonance imaging and computed tomography. Am J Roentgenol 1985; 145: 143–147.

Smith J, Ludwig RL, Marcove RC. Sacrococcygeal chordoma. A clinicoradiological study of 60 patients. Skeletal Radiol 1987; 16: 37–44.

Sze G, Uichanco LS, Brant-Zawadzki MN, Davis RL, Gutin PH, Wilson CG, Norman D, Newton TH. Chordomas: MR imaging. Radiology 1988; 166: 187–191.

Yuh WT, Flickinger FW, Barloon TJ, Montgomery WJ. MR imaging of unusual chordomas. J Comput Assist Tomogr 1988; 12: 30–35.

Metastases

Avrahami E, Tadmor R, Daily O, Hadar H. Early MR demonstration of spinal metastases in patients with normal radiographs and CT and radionuclide bone scans. J Comput Assist Tomogr 1989; 13: 598–602.

Daffner RA, Lupetin AR, Dash N, Deeb ZL, Sefczek RJ, Shapiro RL. MRI in the detection of malignancy infiltration of bone marrow. Am J Roentgenol 1986; 1146: 353–358.

Delbeke D, Powers TA, Sandler MP. Negative scintigraphy with positive magnetic resonance imaging in bone metastases. Skeletal Radiol 1990; 19: 113–116.

Hendrix RW, Rogers LF, Davis TM Jr. Cortical bone metastases. Radiology 1991; 181: 409–413.

Jacobson HG, Poppel MH, Shapiro JH, Grossberger S. The vertebral pedicle sign: a Roentgen finding to differentiate metastatic carcinoma from multiple myeloma. Am J Roentgenol 1958; 80: 817–821.

Ludwig H, Kumpan W, Sinzinger H. Radiography and bone scintigraphy in multiple myeloma: a comparative analysis. Br J Radiol 1982; 55: 173–181.

Rafii M, Firooznia H, Colimbu C, Beranbaum E. CT of skeletal metastasis. Semin Ultrasound Comput Tomogr Magn Reson Imaging 1986; 7: 371–379.

Resnick D, Niwayama C. Skeletal metastases. In: Resnick D, ed. Diagnosis of bone and joint disorders, 3rd ed. Philadelphia: WB Saunders, 1995; 3991–4064.

Schweitzer ME, Levine C, Mitchell DC, Cannon FH, Comella LG. Bull's-eyes and halos: useful MR discriminators of osseous metastases. Radiology 1993; 188: 249–252.

Synovial Chondromatoses

Greenspan A, Azouz EM, Matthews J II, Decarie J-C. Synovial hemangioma: imaging features in eight histologically proved cases, review of the literature, and differential diagnosis. Skeletal Radiol 1995; 24: 583–590.

Hermann C, Abdelwahab IF, Klein MJ, Kenan S, Lewis M. Synovial chondromatosis. Skeletal Radiol 1995; 24: 298–300.

Milgram JW. Synovial osteochondromatosis. A histopathological study of thirty cases. J Bone Joint Surg 1977; 59A: 792–801.

Norman A, Steiner GC. Bone erosion in synovial chondromatosis. Radiology 1986; 161: 749–752.

Tuckman G, Wirth CZ. Synovial osteochondromatosis of the shoulder: MR findings. J Comput Assist Tomogr 1989; 13: 360–361.

Pigmented Villonodular Synovitis

De Beuckeleer L, De Schepper A, De Belder F, Van Goethem J, Marques MCB, Broeckx J, Verstraete J, Vermaut F. Magnetic resonance imaging of localized giant cell tumor of the tendon sheath (MRI of localized GCTTS). Eur Radiol 1997; 7: 198–201.

Jelinek JS, Kransdorf MJ, Utz JA, Hudson-Berry B Jr, Thompson JD, Heekin RD, Radowich MS. Imaging of pigmented villonodular synovitis with emphasis on MR imaging. Am J Roentgenol 1989; 152: 337–342.

Karasick D, Karasick S. Giant cell tumor of tendon sheath: spectrum of radiologic findings. Skeletal Radiol 1992; 21: 219–224.

Mandelbaum BR, Grant TT, Hartzman S, Reicher MA, Flannigan B, Bassett LW, Mirra J, Finerman AM. The use of MRI to assist in the diagnosis of pigmented villonodular synovitis of the knee. Clin Orthop 1988; 231: 135–139.

Rao AS, Vigorita VJ. Pigmented villonodular synovitis (giant-cell tumor of the tendon sheath and synovial membrane). A review of eighty-one cases. J Bone Joint Surg 1984; 66A: 76–94.

Sundaram M, McGuire MH, Fletcher J, Wolverson MK, Heiberg E, Shields JB. Magnetic resonance imaging of lesions of synovial origin. Skeletal Radiol 1986; 15: 110–116.

Synovial Hemangioma

Buetow PC, Kransdorf MJ, Moser RP Jr, Jelinek JS, Berrey BH. Radiologic appearance of intramuscular hemangioma with emphasis on MR imaging. Am J Roentgenol 1990; 154: 563–567.

Ehara S, Son M, Tamakawa Y, Nishida J, Abe M, Hachiya J. Fluid-fluid levels in cavernous hemangioma of soft tissue. Skeletal Radiol 1994; 23: 107–109.

Madewell JE, Sweet DE. Tumors and tumor-like lesions in or about joints. In: Resnick D, ed. Bone and joint imaging. Philadelphia: WB Saunders, 1989; 1184.

Resnick D, Oliphant M. Hemophilia-like arthropathy of the knee associated with cutaneous and synovial hemangiomas. Radiology 1975; 114: 323–326.

Suh J-S, Hwang G, Hahn S-B. Soft tissue hemangiomas: MR manifestations in 23 patients. Skeletal Radiol 1994; 23: 621–625.

Synovial Sarcoma

Ishida T, Iijima T, Moriyama S, Nakamura C, Kitagawa T, Machinami R. Intra-articular calcifying synovial sarcoma mimicking synovial chondromarosis. Skeletal Radiol 1996; 25: 766–769.

Jones BC, Sundaram M, Kransdorf MJ. Synovial sarcoma: MR imaging findings in 34 patients. Am J Roentgenol 1993; 161: 827–830.

Kransdorf MJ, Jelinek JS, Moser RP, Utz JA, Brower AC, Hudson TM, Berrey BH. Soft-tissue masses: diagnosis using MR imaging. Am J Roentgenol 1989; 153: 541–547.

Morton MJ, Berquist TH, McLeod RA, Unni KK, Sim FH. MR imaging of synovial sarcoma. Am J Roentgenol 1991; 156: 337–340.

Synovial Chondrosarcoma

Dahlin DC, Unni KK. Chondrosarcoma. In: Bone Tumors, general aspects and data on 8542 Cases, 4th ed. Springfleld, IL: Charles C Thomas, 1986; 227–259.

Perry BE, McQueen DA, Lin JJ. Synovial chondromatosis with malignant degeneration to chondrosarcoma. Report of a case. J Bone Joint Surg 1988; 70A: 1259–1261.